Pituitary Adenomas

Editors

MANISH K. AGHI
LEWIS S. BLEVINS Jr

NEUROSURGERY
CLINICS OF NORTH AMERICA

www.neurosurgery.theclinics.com

Consulting Editors
RUSSELL R. LONSER
DANIEL K. RESNICK

October 2019 • Volume 30 • Number 4

ELSEVIER

1600 John F. Kennedy Boulevard • Suite 1800 • Philadelphia, Pennsylvania, 19103-2899

http://www.theclinics.com

NEUROSURGERY CLINICS OF NORTH AMERICA Volume 30, Number 4
October 2019 ISSN 1042-3680, ISBN-13: 978-0-323-68168-1

Editor: Stacy Eastman
Developmental Editor: Laura Fisher

Neurosurgery Clinics of North America (ISSN 1042-3680) is published quarterly by Elsevier Inc., 360 Park Avenue South, New York, NY 10010-1710. Months of issue are January, April, July, and October. Business and Editorial Offices: 1600 John F. Kennedy Blvd., Suite 1800, Philadelphia, PA 19103-2899. Customer Service Office: 11830 Westline Industrial Drive, St. Louis, MO 63146. Periodicals postage paid at New York, NY, and additional mailing offices. Subscription prices are $430.00 per year (US individuals), $748.00 per year (US institutions), $470.00 per year (Canadian individuals), $928.00 per year (Canadian institutions), $513.00 per year (international individuals), $928.00 per year (international institutions), $100.00 per year (US students), and $255.00 per year (international and Canadian students). International air speed delivery is included in all *Clinics* subscription prices. All prices are subject to change without notice. **POSTMASTER:** Send address changes to *Neurosurgery Clinics of North America*, Elsevier Periodicals Customer Service, 11830 Westline Industrial Drive, St. Louis, MO 63146. **Customer Service: 1-800-654-2452 (US and Canada). From outside the US and Canada, call: 1-314-453-7041. Fax: 1-314-453-5170. E-mail: JournalsCustomerService-usa@elsevier.com (for print support) and journalsonlinesupport-usa@elsevier.com (for online support).**

Reprints. For copies of 100 or more, of articles in this publication, please contact the Commercial Reprints Department, Elsevier Inc., 360 Park Avenue South, New York, NY 10010-1710. Tel. 212-633-3874; Fax: 212-633-3820; E-mail: reprints@elsevier.com.

Neurosurgery Clinics of North America is covered in *MEDLINE/PubMed (Index Medicus), EMBASE/Excerpta Medica, and Current Contents/Clinical Medicine (CC/CM)*.

Contributors

CONSULTING EDITORS

RUSSELL R. LONSER, MD
Professor and Chair, Department of
Neurological Surgery, The Ohio State
University Wexner Medical Center, Columbus,
Ohio, USA

DANIEL K. RESNICK, MD, MS
Professor and Vice Chairman, Program
Director, Department of Neurosurgery,
University of Wisconsin-Madison School of
Medicine and Public Health, Madison,
Wisconsin, USA

EDITORS

MANISH K. AGHI, MD, PhD
Professor and Vice Chair, Neurosurgery,
University of California, San Francisco,
Director, Center for Minimally Invasive
Skull Base Surgery, California Center for
Pituitary Disorders, San Francisco, California,
USA

LEWIS S. BLEVINS Jr, MD
Professor of Medicine and Neurosurgery,
University of California, San Francisco, Medical
Director, California Center for Pituitary
Disorders, San Francisco, California, USA

AUTHORS

MANISH K. AGHI, MD, PhD
Professor and Vice Chair, Neurosurgery,
University of California, San Francisco,
Director, Center for Minimally Invasive
Skull Base Surgery, California Center for
Pituitary Disorders, San Francisco, California,
USA

ADNAN AJMAL, MD
Department of Internal Medicine and
Endocrinology, St. Joseph's Hospital and
Medical Center, Creighton University
School of Medicine, Phoenix, Arizona,
USA

JOAO PAULO ALMEIDA
Division of Neurosurgery, Toronto Western
Hospital, University of Toronto, Toronto,
Ontario, Canada

GARNI BARKHOUDARIAN, MD
Associate Professor, John Wayne
Cancer Institute, Pacific Neuroscience
Institute, Santa Monica, California,
USA

MARVIN BERGSNEIDER, MD
Department of Neurosurgery, Program
Director, University of California,
Los Angeles, Los Angeles, California,
USA

BEVERLY M.K. BILLER, MD
Neuroendocrine Unit, Neuroendocrine
and Pituitary Tumor Clinical Center,
Massachusetts General Hospital,
Professor of Medicine, Harvard Medical
School, Boston, Massachusetts,
USA

LEWIS S. BLEVINS Jr, MD
Professor of Medicine and Neurosurgery,
University of California, San Francisco,
Medical Director, California Center for
Pituitary Disorders, San Francisco, California,
USA

ANSHU BUTTAN, MD
Department of Medicine, Division of
Endocrinology, Cedars-Sinai Medical Center,
Los Angeles, California, USA

VITOR CASTRO
Division of Neurosurgery, Toronto Western
Hospital, University of Toronto, Toronto,
Ontario, Canada

STEVE S. CHO, BS
Medical Student, Perelman School of
Medicine, University of Pennsylvania,
Philadelphia, Pennsylvania, USA

**RICARDO CORREA, MD, EdD, FACP, FACE
FAPCR, CMQ**
Department of Medicine, Division of
Endocrinology, Diabetes and Metabolism,
Phoenix Veterans Administration Medical
Center, University of Arizona College of
Medicine, Creighton School of Medicine,
Mayo School of Medicine, Phoenix, Arizona,
USA

BHARGAV DESAI, MD
Resident Physician, Department of
Neurological Surgery, University of Virginia
Health Sciences Center, Charlottesville,
Virginia, USA

DANIEL A. DONOHO, MD
Department of Neurosurgery, Brigham and
Women's Hospital, Boston, Massachusetts,
USA

JAMES J. EVANS
Department of Neurological Surgery, Thomas
Jefferson University Hospital, Philadelphia,
Pennsylvania, USA

CLAIRE M. FALTERMEIER, MD, PhD
Resident, Department of Neurological Surgery,
University of California, San Francisco, San
Francisco, California, USA

CHRISTOPHER J. FARRELL, MD
Department of Neurological Surgery, Thomas
Jefferson University Hospital, Philadelphia,
Pennsylvania, USA

JUDD H. FASTENBERG
Department of Otolaryngology–Head and Neck
Surgery, Thomas Jefferson University Hospital,
Philadelphia, Pennsylvania, USA

TOMAS GARZON-MUVDI
Department of Neurological Surgery, Thomas
Jefferson University Hospital, Philadelphia,
Pennsylvania, USA

FRED GENTILI
Division of Neurosurgery, Toronto Western
Hospital, University of Toronto, Toronto,
Ontario, Canada

JOHN A. JANE Jr, MD
Professor of Neurosurgery and Pediatrics,
Department of Neurological Surgery, University
of Virginia Health Sciences Center,
Charlottesville, Virginia, USA

PAMELA S. JONES, MD, MS, MPH
Instructor, Department of Neurosurgery,
Massachusetts General Hospital, Harvard
Medical School, Boston, Massachusetts,
USA

ARISTOTELIS KALYVAS
Division of Neurosurgery, Toronto Western
Hospital, University of Toronto, Toronto,
Ontario, Canada

CLAIRE KAREKEZI
Division of Neurosurgery, Toronto Western
Hospital, University of Toronto, Toronto,
Ontario, Canada; Department of Neurosurgery,
Rwanda Military Hospital, Kigali, Rwanda

DANIEL F. KELLY, MD
Professor, John Wayne Cancer Institute,
Pacific Neuroscience Institute, Santa Monica,
California, USA

WI JIN KIM, MD
Department of Neurosurgery, University of
California, Los Angeles, Los Angeles,
California, USA

EDWARD R. LAWS Jr, MD, FACS
Department of Neurosurgery, Brigham and
Women's Hospital, Boston, Massachusetts,
USA

JOHN Y.K. LEE, MD, MSCE
Assistant Professor, Department of
Neurosurgery, Hospital of the University of
Pennsylvania, Philadelphia, Pennsylvania,
USA

ANDREW S. LITTLE, MD, FAANS, FACS
Department of Neurosurgery, Barrow Pituitary
Center, Barrow Neurological Institute, St.
Joseph's Hospital and Medical Center,
University of Arizona College of Medicine,
Phoenix, Arizona, USA

STEPHEN T. MAGILL, MD, PhD
Resident, Department of Neurological Surgery, University of California, San Francisco, San Francisco, California, USA

ADAM N. MAMELAK, MD, FAANS
Department of Neurosurgery, Cedars-Sinai Medical Center, Los Angeles, California, USA

MIGUEL MARIGIL SANCHEZ, MD, PhD
Division of Neurosurgery, Toronto Western Hospital, University of Toronto, Toronto, Ontario, Canada; Department of Neurosurgery, Skull Base Research Unit, Lariboisière University Hospital, Paris, France

ALEXANDRIA C. MARINO, MD, PhD
Resident Physician, Department of Neurological Surgery, University of Virginia Health Sciences Center, Charlottesville, Virginia, USA

GURSTON G. NYQUIST
Department of Otolaryngology–Head and Neck Surgery, Thomas Jefferson University Hospital, Philadelphia, Pennsylvania, USA

NELSON M. OYESIKU, MD, PhD
Department of Neurosurgery, Emory University, Atlanta, Georgia, USA

GIYARPURAM PRASHANT, MD
Department of Neurosurgery, University of California, Los Angeles, Los Angeles, California, USA

MINDY R. RABINOWITZ
Department of Otolaryngology–Head and Neck Surgery, Thomas Jefferson University Hospital, Philadelphia, Pennsylvania, USA

MARC R. ROSEN
Department of Otolaryngology–Head and Neck Surgery, Thomas Jefferson University Hospital, Philadelphia, Pennsylvania, USA

MARTIN RUTKOWSKI, MD
Open and Endoscopic Skull Base Fellow, Department of Neurosurgery, Keck School of Medicine at USC, University of Southern California, Los Angeles, California, USA

HASSAN SAAD, MD
Department of Neurosurgery, Emory University, Atlanta, Georgia, USA

BROOKE SWEARINGEN, MD
Professor, Department of Neurosurgery, Massachusetts General Hospital, Harvard Medical School, Boston, Massachusetts, USA

DAVIS G. TAYLOR, MD
Resident Physician, Department of Neurological Surgery, University of Virginia Health Sciences Center, Charlottesville, Virginia, USA

NICHOLAS A. TRITOS, MD, DSc
Neuroendocrine Unit, Neuroendocrine and Pituitary Tumor Clinical Center, Massachusetts General Hospital, Associate Professor of Medicine, Harvard Medical School, Boston, Massachusetts, USA

BENJAMIN UY, MD, PhD
Department of Neurosurgery, University of California, Los Angeles, Los Angeles, California, USA

KUMAR VASUDEVAN, MD
Department of Neurosurgery, Emory University, Atlanta, Georgia, USA

CARLOS VELASQUEZ
Division of Neurosurgery, Toronto Western Hospital, University of Toronto, Toronto, Ontario, Canada; Department of Neurological Surgery, Hospital Universitario Marques de Valdecilla and Instituto de Investigacion Marques de Valdecilla (IDIVAL), Santander, Spain

BAYARD WILSON, MD
Department of Neurosurgery, University of California, Los Angeles, Los Angeles, California, USA

KEVIN C.J. YUEN, MD, FRCP (UK), FACE
Department of Neuroendocrinology, Barrow Pituitary Center, Barrow Neurological Institute, St. Joseph's Hospital and Medical Center, University of Arizona College of Medicine, Creighton School of Medicine, Phoenix, Arizona, USA

GABRIEL ZADA, MD, MS
Associate Professor of Neurosurgery, Otolaryngology, and Internal Medicine, Department of Neurosurgery, Keck School of Medicine of USC, University of Southern California, Los Angeles, California, USA

Contents

Pituitary adenomas are benign tumors, but still cause significant morbidity and in some cases increases in mortality. Surgical resection is not without risks, and approximately 40% of adenomas are incompletely resected. Medical therapies such as dopamine agonists, somatostatin analogues, and growth hormone antagonists are associated with numerous side effects. Understanding the molecular biology of pituitary adenomas may yield new therapeutic approaches. Additional studies are needed to help determine which genes or pathways are "drivers" of tumorigenesis and should be therapeutic targets. Further studies may also enable pituitary adenoma stratification to tailor treatment approaches.

Tumor recurrence in pituitary adenomas is as high as 20% after surgery. Conventional neuronavigation and white light visualization are not sufficiently accurate in detecting residual neoplastic tissue. Fluorescence-guided surgery offers accurate, real-time visualization of neoplastic tissue. The authors' group has explored the use of near-infrared imaging, which is superior to visible-light fluorescence in both signal contrast and tissue penetration, in transsphenoidal endoscopic surgeries for pituitary adenomas using 2 techniques: second window indocyanine green, in which indocyanine green passively accumulates in the tumor, and OTL38, which actively targets folate receptors on adenoma cells. This work establishes the foundation of intraoperative near-infrared imaging for fluorescence-guided neurosurgery.

Since the 1990s, MRI scanners have been incorporated into the operating room environment. Studies of the use of intraoperative MRI (iMRI) for pituitary adenomas have shown that images are highly sensitive and specific for residual tumor detection, especially at higher Tesla magnet strengths. Given this accuracy, iMRI also increases the rates of achieving gross total resection (GTR). Owing to the slow-growing nature of pituitary adenomas, comparison of long-term control rates with and without use of iMRI remains to be studied, but the increased rates of GTR with this technology are promising for improved long-term outcomes.

Endoscopic endonasal transsphenoidal approach to the sella (EES) for pituitary adenomas has become standard of care because of its promising outcomes, minimal invasiveness, and popularity among surgeons. Three-dimensional (3D) endoscope technology represents the next step in improving visualization and understanding of surgical anatomy, allowing surgeons to mirror the view offered by a traditional 3D microscope. This article discusses the history and development of 3D endoscopes, addresses theoretic advantages and disadvantages of using these devices for EES, reviews recent studies of EES for adenoma outcomes using 3D endoscopes, examines possible implications for neurosurgical training, and discusses personal experience with 3D devices.

Giant adenomas represent a significant surgical challenge. Although traditionally several transcranial and transsphenoidal microscopic approaches have had a central role in their management, in the last 2 decades here have been increasing reports of the endoscopic endonasal approach for giant adenomas, citing its improved resection rates and lower complication profile. However, its role as the preferred approach has not been fully established and there is currently a paucity of evidence-based recommendations available in the literature. This article reviews the current literature and attempts to define the role and outcomes of the endoscopic endonasal surgical approach for giant pituitary adenomas.

Cavernous sinuses are complex dural venous sinuses that house important neurovascular structures, which often preclude full surgical access for tumor resection. Neuroimaging and anatomic grading scales have corroborated that more invasive tumors are less likely to undergo gross total resection and biochemical remission. Endoscopic approaches are increasingly favored over microsurgical techniques. Direct transcavernous approaches have yielded even greater degrees of resection. Radiosurgery is a powerful adjuvant therapy for residual, recurrent, and/or inaccessible cavernous sinus disease that provides excellent tumor control rates and favorable risk-benefit ratios for the achievement of biochemical remission with minimal endocrine morbidity.

Pituitary apoplexy is a clinical condition with acute-onset headaches, vision loss, and/or pituitary dysfunction associated with a hemorrhagic or infarcted pituitary tumor or cyst. Treatment varies based on clinical presentation, although often urgent or emergent surgical resection is indicated. Conservative treatment strategies tend to be applied for more mild conditions of apoplexy. Overall outcomes may be similar in this less severe cohort. Acute-onset vision loss with apoplexy should be treated with urgent or emergent surgical evacuation of hematoma and resection of tumor when possible.

 Video content accompanies this article at http://www.neurosurgery.theclinics.com.

Pituitary adenomas are a rare but important central nervous system tumor in children. Because of differences in growth and development, the manifestations of pituitary adenomas in children may differ from those seen in adults. Unlike adult patients, the pediatric population more often presents with clinically secretory adenomas. Although medical management is first-line treatment of prolactinomas, transsphenoidal surgery is appropriate for most children with Cushing disease and gigantism. Although some pediatric patients present surgical challenges because of small anatomic dimensions or an incompletely developed sphenoid sinus, transsphenoidal surgery can be safely and effectively undertaken in most children, with low complication rates.

Pituitary adenomas are typically slow-growing benign tumors. However, 50% to 60% of tumors progress following subtotal resection and up to 30% recur after apparent complete resection. Options for treatment of recurrent pituitary adenomas include repeat surgical resection, radiation therapy, and systemic therapies. There is no consensus approach for the management of recurrent pituitary adenomas. This article reviews the natural history of recurrent adenomas and emerging biomarkers predictive of clinical behavior as well as the outcomes associated with the various treatment modalities for these challenging tumors, with an emphasis on the surgical treatment.

Visual signs and symptoms are a common manifestation of pituitary adenomas from compression or ischemia of the optic nerves and optic chiasm. Although bitemporal hemianopsia is a classic presenting visual field deficit, additional visual disturbances can result from these tumors. After endoscopic endonasal pituitary surgery, most patients have improvement in visual symptoms. Preoperative factors including retinal nerve fiber layer thickness, severity of preoperative deficit, duration of visual symptoms, tumor size, extent of resection, and patient age serve as possible predictors of postoperative visual outcomes.

Although removal of pituitary tumors yields excellent surgical outcomes, perturbations in the hypothalamic-pituitary axis are not uncommon. Careful assessment of postoperative hormone status with supplementation or further medical therapy is critical to successful outcomes. Although many centers routinely use perioperative steroids, they can be associated with worse outcomes in the absence of intact preoperative adrenal function or damage to the pituitary gland or stalk during surgery. Postoperative assessment of prolactin, cortisol, and growth hormone can be prognostic of surgical cure. Hormonal axes should be reevaluated routinely several weeks after surgery, because longitudinal monitoring is important for surgical and medical outcomes.

Medical therapy for Cushing disease is primarily used to control hypercortisolism in patients whose disease persists or with recurrent disease after pituitary surgery, including those awaiting the salutary effects of radiation therapy. In can also be used to control hypercortisolism preoperatively, and in patients who decline surgery or whose tumor location is unknown. Steroidogenesis inhibitors, centrally acting agents, and glucocorticoid receptor antagonists are currently available to treat hypercortisolism, and several novel agents are in development. Given the absence of head-to-head clinical trials, choice between treatments has to be individualized based on careful consideration of patient, tumor, and disease characteristics.

Prolactinomas are the most common functional pituitary adenoma. Many prolactinomas can be treated with medication, but all patients should be evaluated at a neuroendocrine center including experienced neurosurgeons trained in transsphenoidal surgery. Surgery for prolactinomas is feasible and can be performed with low morbidity. Patients never previously treated with dopamine agonists should be considered for surgery if they have neurologic deficits, pituitary apoplexy, an uncertain diagnosis, or a significantly cystic prolactinoma. Patients previously treated with dopamine agonists should be considered for surgery in cases of intolerance or resistance. Recurrent and aggressive prolactinomas often require multimodal therapy.

Sodium perturbations are a common complication after pituitary surgery, with hyponatremia being the most frequent. Postoperative assessments should be tailored to the early and late periods, and monitoring sodium perturbations is recommended. Cerebral salt wasting is rare after pituitary surgery, and diagnosis and management can be challenging. Providing patient counseling and close postoperative follow-up is important to effectively manage diabetes insipidus and reduce hospital readmissions due to sodium perturbations.

NEUROSURGERY CLINICS OF NORTH AMERICA

SERIES OF RELATED INTEREST

Neurologic Clinics
http://www.neurologicclinics.com
Neuroimaging Clinics
http://www.neuroimaging.theclinics.com/

THE CLINICS ARE AVAILABLE ONLINE!
Access your subscription at:
www.theclinics.com

Preface
Introduction to Pituitary Adenomas

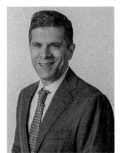 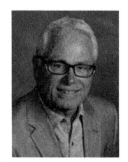

Manish K. Aghi, MD, PhD   Lewis S. Blevins Jr, MD
Editors

Pituitary adenomas are the third most common intracranial neoplasm in adults, accounting for about 10% of all intracranial tumors. Pituitary adenomas can be functional adenomas that cause hormone hypersecretion and associated symptoms or nonfunctional adenomas that do not secrete excess hormones. Either of these 2 types of pituitary adenomas can cause symptoms of mass effect, such as vision loss, hypopituitarism, or headaches. Pituitary adenomas are occasionally detected on imaging studies performed for unrelated reasons. These tumors are commonly referred to as "pituitary incidentaloma" as the detection was incidental and unexpected in the evaluation of some other process.

We are at an exciting time in the management of pituitary adenomas as we stand at the precipice of landmark innovations in our molecular understanding of these tumors and their endocrine and neurosurgical management. As such, we are excited to bring you this issue of *Neurosurgery Clinics of North America* devoted to pituitary adenomas. Specifically, the goals of this issue are to offer the reader a comprehensive overview of the latest advances in the management of pituitary adenomas. Specifically, we present an overview of the molecular biology of pituitary adenomas, concerns specific to functional adenomas (Cushing disease, prolactinomas), neurosurgical nuances related to the management of challenging pituitary adenomas (those invading the cavernous sinus, giant adenomas,

and pituitary apoplexy), neurosurgical adjuncts of value in pituitary adenoma surgery (intraoperative MRI, 3D endoscopy, and fluorescent dyes enabling tumor visualization), postoperative issues of concern (hormonal function and sodium perturbations), and management of recurrent nonfunctional adenomas.

These contributions are presented by some of the world's foremost experts in endocrinology and neurosurgery. We hope the combined perspective of these experts will make this issue a valuable resource for physicians caring for patients with pituitary adenomas.

Manish K. Aghi, MD, PhD
Department of Neurosurgery
University of California, San Francisco
Center for Minimally Invasive Skull Base Surgery
California Center for Pituitary Disorders
505 Parnassus Avenue, Room M779
San Francisco, CA 94143-0112, USA

Lewis S. Blevins Jr, MD
Department of Neurosurgery
University of California, San Francisco
California Center for Pituitary Disorders
400 Parnassus Avenue Room A-808
San Francisco, CA 94143-0350, USA

E-mail addresses:
manish.aghi@ucsf.edu (M.K. Aghi)
lewis.blevins@ucsf.edu (L.S. Blevins)

neurosurgery.theclinics.com

Molecular Biology of Pituitary Adenomas

Claire M. Faltermeier, MD, PhD[a], Stephen T. Magill, MD, PhD[a], Lewis S. Blevins Jr, MD[a,b], Manish K. Aghi, MD, PhD[a],*

KEYWORDS

- Pituitary adenomas • Somatotroph adenomas • Corticotroph adenomas • Lactotroph adenomas
- Thyrotroph adenomas • Gonadotroph adenomas • Null cell adenomas • Molecular biology

KEY POINTS

- Despite the benign nature of pituitary adenomas, they still cause significant morbidity and can increase mortality. A better understanding of the molecular pathogenesis of pituitary adenomas may yield new therapeutic approaches.
- The pathogenesis of pituitary adenomas is multifactorial with genetic mutations, alterations in gene transcription, and epigenetics interacting to promote tumorigenesis.
- Fewer than 5% of patients with pituitary adenomas have familial syndromes with associated germline mutations in MEN1, AIP, and PRKAR1A. Although rare, these mutations highlight that activation of proliferation pathways are important in pituitary tumorigenesis.
- Somatic mutations in GNAS1 and USP8 likely contribute to the development of somatotroph and corticotroph adenomas; however, the precise role of these mutations in tumorigenesis remains unknown.
- In adenomas without recurrent genetic alterations, differential protein expression or epigenetic alterations may be helpful to stratify patients with aggressive versus nonaggressive tumors. This information may be useful for determining the need for adjuvant therapy.

INTRODUCTION

Pituitary adenomas are the second most common intracranial tumor.[1,2] The incidence of pituitary adenomas is increasing, likely due to improved methods of radiographic detection.[2] Pituitary adenomas are classified based on immunohistochemical staining of the hormone content and primary transcription factor in the tumor.[3] Functioning tumors include somatotroph (growth hormone [GH] secreting, Pit1+), lactotroph (prolactin [PRL] secreting, Pit-1+), thyrotroph (thyroid-stimulating hormone [TSH] secreting, Pit-1, GATA-2 +), corticotroph (adrenocorticotropic hormone [ACTH] secreting, Tpit+), gonadotroph (β-follicle-stimulating hormone [FSH], β-luteinizing hormone [LH], SF-1, GATA-2, ER-α +), plurihormonal, and null cell.[3] Null cell adenomas do not secrete hormones and are negative for expression of lineage transcription factors.[3]

Treatment of pituitary adenomas is dependent on tumor subtype. Prolactinomas are initially treated with dopaminergic therapies. For other subtypes, first-line therapy is transsphenoidal resection through either microscopic or endoscopic techniques. Risks of surgery include but are not limited to, hypopituitarism, cerebrospinal fluid leakage, or meningitis. Unfortunately, not all

Disclosure Statement: The authors have nothing to disclose.
[a] Department of Neurological Surgery, University of California, San Francisco, 505 Parnassus Avenue Suite M779, San Francisco, CA 94143-0112, USA; [b] Medicine (Endocrinology), University of California, San Francisco, San Francisco, CA, USA
* Corresponding author.
E-mail address: manish.aghi@ucsf.edu
; @StephenTMagill1 (S.T.M.); @manishkaghi (M.K.A.)

Neurosurg Clin N Am 30 (2019) 391–400
https://doi.org/10.1016/j.nec.2019.05.001

tumors can be completely resected, and many patients will require additional therapeutic modalities. For patients with somatotroph tumors, medical therapies target the GH receptor or somatostatin receptors with somatostatin receptor ligands or GH receptor antagonists. However, these therapies are not 100% effective and have side effects.

Despite the benign nature of most pituitary adenomas, they still lead to significant morbidity and can increase mortality. The clinical syndromes of acromegaly and Cushing disease have numerous medical complications, such as hypertension, cardiac disease, and diabetes, often leading to premature death.[4] Mass effect from pituitary tumors can cause visual impairment by compression of the optic apparatus. Effective long-term treatment is also an issue, as 40% of tumors cannot be completely resected due to invasion into surrounding structures, and tumors that undergo gross-total resection have a 10% to 30% risk of recurrence.[5] These issues highlight the need for new therapeutic approaches that are more effective.

Improving our understanding of the molecular pathogenesis of pituitary adenomas may yield novel therapeutic targets. Although pituitary adenomas are likely monoclonal in origin, ubiquitous driver mutations have yet to be identified.[6] One hypothesis is that a single genetic mutation leads to tumor development. Although rare, germline mutations in genes such as multiple endocrine neoplasia type 1 (MEN1) and AIP have been associated with pituitary adenomas in the absence of other associated genetic changes; however, the precise roles of these mutations are unclear. In fact, the pathogenesis of most pituitary adenomas is likely multifactorial with genetic mutations, alterations in gene transcription, and epigenetics interacting to promote tumorigenesis. This review focuses on understanding the current state of the molecular biology of pituitary adenomas, stratified by histologic type, with an emphasis on the genetic, transcriptomic, and epigenetic alterations within each subtype. We also highlight the translational relevance of these alterations.

SOMATOTROPH ADENOMAS

Somatotroph adenomas represent 15% to 20% of all pituitary adenomas[7] (**Fig. 1**), and cause the clinical syndrome of acromegaly through GH hypersecretion. Patients with acromegaly have morbidity and premature mortality due to metabolic, pulmonary, and cardiovascular complications. First-line therapy is surgical resection, with medical therapy using somatostatin analogues,

dopamine agonists, and GH receptor antagonists reserved for subtotal resections or recurrent disease.[8] Not all somatotroph adenomas behave similarly. Correlation of histology and clinical course has shown that densely granulated somatotroph adenomas, tend to be smaller and more responsive to somatostatin inhibitors,[9] whereas sparsely granulated somatotroph adenomas are more likely to be larger and resistant to somatostatin inhibitors.[9] However, the molecular mechanisms that lead to the initiation of somatotroph adenomas, and differences in clinical behavior are incompletely understood.

Familial syndromes are associated with fewer than 5% of somatotroph adenomas.[8] Although rare, germline mutations occurring in these syndromes may provide insight into pathways important in the formation of somatotroph adenomas. Inactivating mutations in the tumor-suppressor gene, PRKAR1A (protein kinase cAMP-dependent type 1 regulatory subunit alpha) leads to Carney complex, a syndrome associated with hyperpigmentation, cardiac myxomas, and somatotroph adenomas.[10] Inactivation of PRKAR1A leads to cell proliferation through increasing cAMP levels, which activates the cAMP-dependent kinase, protein kinase A (PKA).[11] The syndrome "familial isolated pituitary adenoma" or FIPA, is an autosomal dominant condition in which pituitary adenomas are the only tumor type affected patients are predisposed to form, with most affected families having at least 3 family members with pituitary adenomas. Most patients with FIPA have somatotroph adenomas, and genetic profiling has shown that 20% of these tumors have inactivating mutations in either aryl hydrocarbon receptor interacting gene (AIP) or duplication of G-coupled protein receptor 101 (GPR101).[12] Mutations in AIP and duplication in GPR101, similar to mutations in PRKAR1A, also lead to elevated cAMP and increased cell proliferation.[12,13]

Somatic mutations affect a much larger proportion of patients with somatotroph adenomas. Approximately 40% of somatotroph adenomas carry activating mutations in the G-protein alpha subunit (G_s-α), GNAS1. Similar to the germline mutations described previously, somatic GNAS1 mutations in tumor cells lead to elevated cAMP levels, PKA activation, and GH secretion.[14,15] It remains unknown if GNAS1 mutations are the initiating event in somatotroph tumorigenesis, or if they are a secondary event contributing to maintenance of tumor growth. The clinical significance of GNAS1 mutations in somatotroph adenomas is also unclear. A retrospective study of 60 somatotroph tumors with GNAS1 mutations, found that

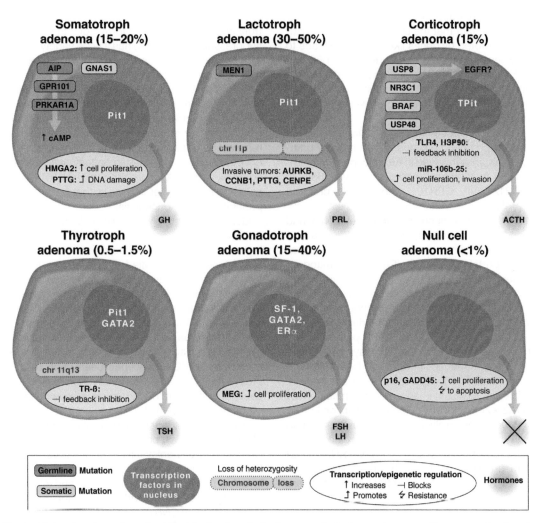

Fig. 1. Molecular alterations described in the 6 pathologic types of pituitary adenomas. Shown are the 6 patho-logic types of pituitary adenomas (somatotroph, lactotroph, corticotroph, thyrotroph, gonadotroph, and null cell), what percentage of total adenomas they represent, and the molecular alterations that have been described in them. miRNA, microRNA.

these tumors had higher preoperative insulin like growth factor-1 (IGF-1) levels and tended to be smaller tumors than GNAS1 wild-type tumors. However, there were no differences in proliferation, response to somatostatin therapy, or recurrence after surgery between patients with GNAS1 mutant or wild-type tumors.[16] Cytogenetic profiling of somatotroph tumors found that GNAS1 wild-type tumors had increased copy-number alterations compared with GNAS1 mutant tumors.[17] This study suggests that, in GNAS1 wild-type tumors, genomic instability may be an alternative pathway to achieve the elevated cAMP levels, PKA activation, and GH secretion found in GNAS1-mutated tumors.

Nonmutated genes also have been implicated in somatotroph tumorigenesis. Transgenic mice with overexpression of the high-mobility AT-hook protein, HMGA2 develop GH-secreting and PRL-secreting adenomas.[18] HMGA2 has numerous functions, but its role in pituitary tumorigenesis is likely to drive cell cycle progression by inhibiting the cell cycle inhibitor pRB and enhancing E2F1 activity.[19,20] Overexpression of the pituitary tumor transforming protein (PTTG) is found in almost all pituitary adenomas, but GH-secreting adenomas often have the highest expression.[21] PTTG overexpression induces cellular transformation in vitro, aneuploidy, and DNA damage by regulating the segregation of sister chromatids during mitosis. Despite expression of genes promoting cell cycle dysregulation, somatotroph adenomas rarely progress to malignancy. This may be because the cell cycle–promoting effects of the altered genes in somatotroph adenomas are counteracted by the fact that the DNA damage and aneuploidy promoted by genes like PTTG also leads to cell cycle arrest through upregulation of p53 and p21.[22] Furthermore, GH itself has been shown to protect quiescent and senescent somatotroph cells from apoptosis, enabling slow-growing adenomas to thrive.[23]

Research investigating the pathogenesis of somatotroph adenomas has uncovered key pathways and genes involved in tumorigenesis with implications for potential therapeutics. Mutations in PRKAR1A, AIP, GPR101, and GNAS1 promote cell proliferation by increasing intracellular cAMP. In other cancers, such as uveal melanoma and appendiceal carcinoma,[24,25] GNAS1 mutations are thought to promote tumorigenesis by activation of protein kinase C (PKC), and mitogen-activated protein kinase (MAPK) signaling. Inhibition of these pathways has decreased uveal melanoma growth in vitro.[26] It is unknown whether the GNAS1 mutation in somatotroph adenomas leads to activation of the PKC and MAPK pathways, but if it does, targeting of these pathways could have potential therapeutic relevance. Both HMGA2 and PTTG are also attractive treatment targets. Multiple studies have shown that inhibition of HMGA2 expression by microRNA-33b or Let-7c can block cell proliferation and metastasis in breast cancer and squamous cell carcinoma,[27,28] which raises the possibility that small RNA-based therapeutics may be a potential treatment avenue, but this has not been investigated for pituitary tumors.

LACTOTROPH ADENOMAS

Lactotroph adenomas are the most common type of functioning pituitary adenomas, representing 30% to 50% of all adenomas (see **Fig. 1**).[3] The most common morphologic variants of lactotroph adenomas are sparsely granulated lactotroph adenoma (SGLA), densely granulated lactotroph adenoma, and acidophil stem cell adenoma. SGLA and acidophil stem cell adenomas tend to be more aggressive and less responsive to dopamine agonists.[5] First-line therapy is medical management with dopamine agonists, such as bromocriptine or cabergoline, which inhibit prolactin release and cause a reduction in tumor size; however, these medications are often not tolerated by patients because of side effects.

As with somatotroph adenomas, prolactinomas are rarely caused by germline mutations. The most common genetic syndrome associated with prolactinomas is MEN1, a syndrome in which patients develop parathyroid, pancreatic, and pituitary tumors.[12] Mutations in the MEN1 gene lead to a truncated or inactive form of the tumor-suppressor menin, which has a wide variety of molecular functions.[12] The mechanism by which loss of menin promotes tumorigenesis is not fully understood, but one role is to promote cell proliferation by downregulation of cell cycle inhibitors.[29] MEN1-associated prolactinomas tend to be clinically aggressive, and approximately 45% are resistant to dopamine therapies.[30] Prolactinomas have also been diagnosed in patients with Carney complex and FIPA, implicating AIP and PRKAR1A as being part of other pathways that converge on prolactinoma tumorigenesis.[12]

Genetic profiling of sporadic prolactinomas has not identified any common recurrent mutations; however, chromosomal losses and rearrangements have been identified. Genomic hybridization found that aggressive prolactinomas are associated with loss of chromosome 11p.[31] Some of the genes that are lost due to 11p deletion are associated with inhibiting cell cycle progression and cell invasion, which may explain why these tumors are more aggressive. Similar to GH-secreting adenomas, HMGA2 also has been implicated in prolactinomas. HMGA2 is overexpressed by gene amplification or structural rearrangements of the gene locus on chromosome 12.[32]

Transcriptomic analysis of prolactinomas has identified genes associated with clinical behavior. Comparison of noninvasive with invasive tumors found that invasive tumors had upregulation of invasion-related genes (ADAMTS6 and CRMP1) and genes associated with proliferation, such as PTTG, ASK, CCNB1, AURKB, and CENPE.[33] Another study of 94 patients with prolactinomas identified many of the same genes (ADAMTS6, CRMP1, PTTG, ASK, CCNB1, AURKB, and CENPE), which were associated with tumor recurrence or aggressive behavior.[34] Two of these proteins, aurora kinase B (AURKB) and cyclin B1 (CCNB1) have been implicated in numerous cancers, promoting cell proliferation and survival.[35–37]

Research on prolactinomas has identified key pathways that promote cell proliferation. Although there are likely additional mechanisms, significant pathways include downregulation of cell cycle inhibitors or inactivation of tumor-suppressor genes, such as MEN1. Multiple genes have been identified that are upregulated in aggressive tumors, but functional studies investigating their role in tumorigenesis are lacking. Inhibitors targeting one of these proteins, aurora kinase B, have shown to inhibit tumor growth and promote apoptosis in other cancers,[36] and could be considered as a potential option in some prolactinomas. Although dopamine agonists are effective in treating most prolactinomas, investigations studying pathways that drive the growth of large incompletely resectable tumors that are resistant or not responsive to dopamine agonists may yield additional therapeutic targets.[38]

CORTICOTROPH ADENOMAS

Corticotroph adenomas represent approximately 15% of functioning pituitary adenomas (see Fig. 1). Most corticotroph adenomas, but not all, secrete ACTH, leading to Cushing disease. There are 3 histologic subtypes: densely granulated corticotroph adenoma (DGCA), sparsely granulated corticotroph adenoma (SGCA), and Crooke cell adenoma, which has cytoplasmic accumulation of cytokeratin filaments.[39] Twenty percent of these adenomas do not secrete ACTH and are considered "silent" corticotroph adenomas.[40] The standard of care is surgery, which leads to remission in 65% to 90% of cases.

There are no common germline mutations associated with corticotroph adenomas; however, somatic mutations have been identified in 20% to 60% of patients. The most common is an activating mutation in the ubiquitin specific peptidase 8 enzyme, USP8, which functions to remove ubiquitin from proteins thereby preventing their degradation.[41,42] USP8 may promote tumorigenesis by deubiquitinating the epidermal growth factor receptor (EGFR), leading to increased cell proliferation and invasiveness.[43] USP8 also has been implicated in increasing the production of the precursor of ACTH, pro-opiomelanocortin (POMC), through EGFR-ERK1/2 signaling.[44] Clinical studies show that USP8 mutant adenomas are more common in women, and are more likely to achieve remission after surgical resection.[45] In USP8 wild-type tumors, mutations have been identified in the glucocorticoid receptor gene, NR3C1,[46] the deubiquitinase USP48, and the serine/threonine kinase BRAF.[47] The function of the NR3C1 mutation is unknown, but it may prevent feedback inhibition by ACTH. Finally, a recent study identified mutations in USP48 and BRAF that increase the activity of nuclear factor-κB and c-fos–mediated ACTH transcription, thereby leading to the formation of corticotrophic adenomas.[47] Significantly, the BRAF mutation is at V600 E, which is the most commonly found mutation in malignant melanoma and has inhibitors approved by the Food and Drug Administration on the market.

Epigenetic mechanisms have been implicated in corticotroph adenoma growth and resistance to apoptosis. DNA methylation profiling of 13 ACTH adenomas found hypomethylation of the POMC gene, and no differences in the methylation profile between USP8 mutant and wild-type tumors.[48] Furthermore, treatment of corticotroph adenoma cells with a histone deacetylase inhibitor lead to apoptosis, through decreased LXR-dependent POMC transcription.[49] MicroRNAs have been associated with clinical behavior in patients with corticotrophic adenoma. In Crooke cell adenoma the miR-106b~25 cluster was found to be highly expressed[50] and has been associated with increased cell proliferation and invasiveness though downregulation of phosphatase and tensin homolog (PTEN) and activation of PI3K/AKT signaling.[51]

Mechanisms of glucocorticoid receptor (GR) resistance to feedback inhibition are also important in the pathogenesis of corticotroph adenomas. In nontumorigenic corticotroph cells, binding of steroids to GR leads to translocation of the receptor to the nucleus and inhibition of POMC transcription. Testicular orphan nuclear receptor 4 (TLR4) is overexpressed in corticotroph adenoma and promotes transcription of POMC through a GR-independent manner.[52] Another mechanism of resistance to GR feedback inhibition is through overexpression of the heat-shock protein 90 (HSP90). GR relies on HSP90 for proper folding; however, corticotroph adenomas have overexpression of HSP90, leading to continued GR-HSP90 complexes, and inhibition of GR-DNA binding.[53] Furthermore, inhibition of HSP90 decreased plasma ACTH levels by reactivating GR-mediated feedback inhibition.

Research on corticotroph adenomas has identified multiple pathways involved in tumorigenesis that are therapeutically targetable. USP8 mutant tumors, if associated with EGFR activation, may be susceptible to EGFR inhibition. In USP8 wild-type tumors that have a BRAF V600 E mutation, BRAF inhibitors that are currently on the market are a very attractive therapeutic option. BRAF[V600E] inhibitors have produced durable clinical responses in metastatic melanoma and non–small-cell lung cancer, and clinical trials are ongoing targeting BRAF[V600E] in central nervous system tumors.[54–56] However, like EGFR, studies investigating the functional role of BRAF[V600E] mutations in corticotroph adenomas are needed. Perhaps the most promising therapeutic approach is targeting resistance to negative feedback. Inhibition of MEK1/2 and HSP90 in murine models potently inhibits tumor growth and decreases ACTH levels.

THYROTROPINOMAS

TSH-secreting adenomas are the least common type of pituitary adenomas, representing between

0.5% and 1.5%[3] (see **Fig. 1**) of pituitary adenomas. Histologically, they are identified by variable expression of β-TSH and nuclear expression of Pit-1.[3] Thyrotropinomas on presentation are usually macroadenomas and have extrasellar extension.[57] As a result, only between one-third and one-half of patients are cured by surgical resection alone and most require additional medical therapy.[57–59]

Unlike other pituitary adenomas, thyrotropinomas are not associated with genetic syndromes or common somatic mutations. Several cases have been identified with loss of heterozygosity of 11q13, most commonly found in patients with MEN1; however, these tumors had a wild-type *MEN1* gene, suggesting that menin does not play a role in thyrotropinoma pathogenesis.[60] Whole-exome sequencing was performed on 8 thyrotropinomas, demonstrating a low mutation burden and lack of recurrent mutations.[61]

Although common genetic mutations do not appear to play a role, multiple studies have implicated thyroid and somatostatin receptors in TSH-adenoma tumorigenesis. Patients with thyrotropinomas have elevated thyroid hormones in the setting of an elevated TSH, suggesting that the tumors have impaired negative feedback. This impairment may be though altered expression of the thyroid receptor (TR). Mice expressing a mutant form of TR-beta, which lacks the binding domain for thyroid hormone, develop spontaneous pituitary adenomas.[62] Alternative splicing and mutations of the TR receptor impairing negative feedback by thyroid hormone have been found in a few cases of human thyrotropinomas.[63,64]

Perhaps the most clinically relevant finding in thyrotropinomas is that somatostatin inhibits TSH secretion by binding to somatostatin receptors 2 and 5.[65,66] Somatostatin analogues suppress TSH secretion in 90% of patients and can lead to tumor shrinkage[67,68]; however, because of the side effects of somatostatin inhibitors, first-line therapy of thyrotropinomas with somatostatin inhibitors is not widely accepted.[69]

Due to their rarity, studies on the biology of thyrotropinomas are limited by low numbers and the lack of cell lines/models in the laboratory. Although genetic mutations cannot be ruled out as causative mechanisms of tumor growth, they are uncommon. Given the low mutation burden of these tumors, epigenetic studies may yield insights into tumor biology. The elegant studies on showing how alterations in the TR can affect negative feedback on TSH expression have led to another mechanism of thyrotropinoma tumor growth, although these changes seem to be uncommon. The promising clinical responses to somatostatin inhibitors suggests that this pathway is linked to tumor growth.

GONADOTROPH ADENOMAS

Gonadotroph adenomas compromise 15% to 40% of pituitary adenomas (see **Fig. 1**)[70]; however, functioning gonadotroph adenomas, which secrete FSH and LH, are rare. Because most gonadotroph adenomas are nonfunctioning, the most common presentation is due to tumor mass effect. Before 2017, most biological studies on nonfunctioning gonadotroph adenomas were combined with null cell and other nonfunctioning adenomas.[3] As a result, there are few data that specifically study gonadotroph adenomas.

Whole-exome sequencing of 7 nonfunctioning gonadotroph adenomas found a total of 25 mutations, but none of these mutations was recurrent.[71] Transcriptional analysis of fast versus slow-growing nonfunctioning gonadotroph adenomas found that fast-growing adenomas had high expression of genes related to invasiveness.[72] The noncoding RNA MEG, which regulates p53 gene expression, was found to be downregulated by methylation in a series of functioning gonadotroph adenomas.[73,74] Mechanistically, downregulation of MEG is thought to promote cell proliferation. However, as often occurs with adenomas, excessive cell proliferation is counteracted by other changes that slow proliferation. For gonadotroph adenomas, the proliferation driven by downregulated MEG is thought to be countered by high expression of antiproliferative genes p27/p16.[75]

Given the recent reclassification of null cell adenomas to exclude nonfunctioning gonadotroph adenomas, we hope that future studies will provide more insight into the specific mechanisms of gonadotroph adenoma growth and raise potential therapeutic targets for this subset of tumors that is currently managed with surgery and radiation.

NULL CELL ADENOMAS

Null cell adenomas are defined by the World Health Organization (WHO) 2017 classification as has having no evidence of lineage differentiation either by transcription factors or hormones (see **Fig. 1**).[3] The incidence of null cell adenomas is likely less than 1% of all pituitary adenomas,[76] as before 2017 null cell adenomas were defined as "nonfunctioning" by lack of hormone expression, but not transcription factor expression. As a result, there are many gonadotroph adenomas (negative for FSH and LH, but positive for transcription factors SF-1, GATA2, or ERa) that were previously classified as "null cell adenomas." In an analysis of 147 "nonfunctioning" pituitary adenomas that were negative for hormone expression, only 47 were negative for lineage transcription factor expression and thus considered to be true null cell adenomas.[77] Given the recent change in the pathologic classification of null cell adenomas, there is limited literature investigating the molecular biology of these tumors. We briefly review our current state of knowledge of nonfunctioning adenomas, and hope that subsequent studies will build on these results to further define null cell adenomas.

A study performed before the 2017 WHO classification using whole-exome sequencing found no recurrent mutations in nonfunctioning adenomas,[71] but it is unclear if these tumors would have represented null cell adenomas using the current criteria. Sporadic mutations have been identified in PDGF-D, ZAK, and PIK3CA.[71,78] Both PDGF-D and PIK3CA have potent effects on cell proliferation and invasion; however, their precise role in pituitary tumorigenesis is unclear.[79,80] Epigenetic regulation also has been implicated in nonfunctioning adenomas. Methylation of tumor suppressors p16 and GADD45 are thought to promote cell cycle proliferation and resistance to apoptosis.[81,82] At a transcriptional level, downregulation of the transforming growth factor-beta pathway by microRNAs targeting Smad proteins may play a role in nonfunctioning tumor cell growth.[83]

SUMMARY

The mechanisms underlying pituitary tumor pathogenesis are multifactorial, and involve interactions among mutated genes, dysregulated protein expression, and epigenetic alterations. Regardless of tumor subtype, most alterations seem to contribute to increased cell proliferation. Increased expression in cAMP in somatotroph adenomas, loss of genes on chromosome 11p in prolactinomas, and downregulation of noncoding RNAs in gonadotroph adenomas all lead to increased cell proliferation. However, targeting pathways such as cAMP-mediated cell proliferation is unlikely to be successful due to the adverse effect on normal cells. In addition, because most pituitary adenomas are generally slow-growing tumors and often never recur after complete resection, new therapeutics need to have virtually no toxicity for them to be used broadly. An ideal target would be tumor specific and block a "driver" of tumor growth. Mutant GNAS1, USP8, and BRAF may be ideal targets for corticotroph and somatotroph adenomas; however, laboratory studies are still ongoing to determine whether these mutations are the actual drivers of tumor growth. For tumors without known driver mutations, identifying new therapeutic targets remains a challenge. Future efforts will need to build off precise molecular classification of each adenoma type and the correlation of adenoma subtype with clinical behavior. Hopefully, this will allow identification of what makes some tumors within a single adenoma type more aggressive and prone to recurrence and further our understanding of the biology of each adenoma subtype, which will guide us to improved targeted therapeutics.

REFERENCES

1. Fernandez A, Karavitaki N, Wass JA. Prevalence of pituitary adenomas: a community-based, cross-sectional study in Banbury (Oxfordshire, UK). Clin Endocrinol 2010;72(3):377–82.
2. Ostrom QT, Gittleman H, Truitt G, et al. CBTRUS statistical report: primary brain and other central nervous system tumors diagnosed in the United States in 2011-2015. Neuro Oncol 2018;20(suppl_4):iv1–86.
3. Mete O, Lopes MB. Overview of the 2017 WHO classification of pituitary tumors. Endocr Pathol 2017; 28(3):228–43.
4. Jane JA Jr, Laws ER Jr. The surgical management of pituitary adenomas in a series of 3,093 patients. J Am Coll Surg 2001;193(6):651–9.
5. Meij BP, Lopes MB, Ellegala DB, et al. The long-term significance of microscopic dural invasion in 354 patients with pituitary adenomas treated with transsphenoidal surgery. J Neurosurg 2002;96(2):195–208.
6. Herman V, Fagin J, Gonsky R, et al. Clonal origin of pituitary adenomas. J Clin Endocrinol Metab 1990; 71(6):1427–33.
7. Kiseljak-Vassiliades K, Carlson NE, Borges MT, et al. Growth hormone tumor histological subtypes predict response to surgical and medical therapy. Endocrine 2015;49(1):231–41.
8. Melmed S. Pituitary medicine from discovery to patient-focused outcomes. J Clin Endocrinol Metab 2016;101(3):769–77.
9. Syro LV, Rotondo F, Ramirez A, et al. Progress in the diagnosis and classification of pituitary adenomas. Front Endocrinol (Lausanne) 2015;6:97.
10. Kirschner LS, Carney JA, Pack SD, et al. Mutations of the gene encoding the protein kinase A type I-alpha regulatory subunit in patients with the Carney complex. Nat Genet 2000;26(1):89–92.
11. Correa R, Salpea P, Stratakis CA. Carney complex: an update. Eur J Endocrinol 2015;173(4):M85–97.
12. Caimari F, Korbonits M. Novel genetic causes of pituitary adenomas. Clin Cancer Res 2016;22(20):5030–42.

13. Tuominen I, Heliovaara E, Raitila A, et al. AIP inactivation leads to pituitary tumorigenesis through defective Galphai-cAMP signaling. Oncogene 2015;34(9):1174–84.

14. Vallar L, Spada A, Giannattasio G. Altered Gs and adenylate cyclase activity in human GH-secreting pituitary adenomas. Nature 1987;330(6148):566–8.

15. Melmed S. Acromegaly pathogenesis and treatment. J Clin Invest 2009;119(11):3189–202.

16. Freda PU, Chung WK, Matsuoka N, et al. Analysis of GNAS mutations in 60 growth hormone secreting pituitary tumors: correlation with clinical and pathological characteristics and surgical outcome based on highly sensitive GH and IGF-I criteria for remission. Pituitary 2007;10(3):275–82.

17. Hage M, Viengchareun S, Brunet E, et al. Genomic alterations and complex subclonal architecture in sporadic GH-secreting pituitary adenomas. J Clin Endocrinol Metab 2018;103(5):1929–39.

18. Fedele M, Battista S, Kenyon L, et al. Overexpression of the HMGA2 gene in transgenic mice leads to the onset of pituitary adenomas. Oncogene 2002;21(20):3190–8.

19. Fedele M, Visone R, De Martino I, et al. HMGA2 induces pituitary tumorigenesis by enhancing E2F1 activity. Cancer Cell 2006;9(6):459–71.

20. Fedele M, Pierantoni GM, Visone R, et al. E2F1 activation is responsible for pituitary adenomas induced by HMGA2 gene overexpression. Cell Div 2006;1:17.

21. Hunter JA, Skelly RH, Aylwin SJ, et al. The relationship between pituitary tumour transforming gene (PTTG) expression and in vitro hormone and vascular endothelial growth factor (VEGF) secretion from human pituitary adenomas. Eur J Endocrinol 2003;148(2):203–11.

22. Chesnokova V, Zonis S, Kovacs K, et al. p21(Cip1) restrains pituitary tumor growth. Proc Natl Acad Sci U S A 2008;105(45):17498–503.

23. Chesnokova V, Zhou C, Ben-Shlomo A, et al. Growth hormone is a cellular senescence target in pituitary and nonpituitary cells. Proc Natl Acad Sci U S A 2013;110(35):E3331–9.

24. Wilson CH, McIntyre RE, Arends MJ, et al. The activating mutation R201C in GNAS promotes intestinal tumourigenesis in Apc(Min/+) mice through activation of Wnt and ERK1/2 MAPK pathways. Oncogene 2010;29(32):4567–75.

25. Ang C, Stollman A, Zhu H, et al. Clinical benefit from trametinib in a patient with appendiceal adenocarcinoma with a GNAS R201H mutation. Case Rep Oncol 2017;10(2):548–52.

26. Chen X, Wu Q, Tan L, et al. Combined PKC and MEK inhibition in uveal melanoma with GNAQ and GNA11 mutations. Oncogene 2014;33(39):4724–34.

27. Lin Y, Liu AY, Fan C, et al. MicroRNA-33b inhibits breast cancer metastasis by targeting HMGA2, SALL4 and Twist1. Sci Rep 2015;5:9995.

28. Hou B, Ishinaga H, Midorikawa K, et al. Let-7c inhibits migration and epithelial-mesenchymal transition in head and neck squamous cell carcinoma by targeting IGF1R and HMGA2. Oncotarget 2018; 9(10):8927–40.

29. Gillam MP, Nimbalkar D, Sun L, et al. MEN1 tumorigenesis in the pituitary and pancreatic islet requires Cdk4 but not Cdk2. Oncogene 2015;34(7):932–8.

30. Trouillas J, Labat-Moleur F, Sturm N, et al. Pituitary tumors and hyperplasia in multiple endocrine neoplasia type 1 syndrome (MEN1): a case-control study in a series of 77 patients versus 2509 non-MEN1 patients. Am J Surg Pathol 2008;32(4):534–43.

31. Wierinckx A, Roche M, Raverot G, et al. Integrated genomic profiling identifies loss of chromosome 11p impacting transcriptomic activity in aggressive pituitary PRL tumors. Brain Pathol 2011;21(5): 533–43.

32. Fedele M, Palmieri D, Fusco A. HMGA2: a pituitary tumour subtype-specific oncogene? Mol Cell Endocrinol 2010;326(1–2):19–24.

33. Wierinckx A, Auger C, Devauchelle P, et al. A diagnostic marker set for invasion, proliferation, and aggressiveness of prolactin pituitary tumors. Endocr Relat Cancer 2007;14(3):887–900.

34. Raverot G, Wierinckx A, Dantony E, et al. Prognostic factors in prolactin pituitary tumors: clinical, histological, and molecular data from a series of 94 patients with a long postoperative follow-up. J Clin Endocrinol Metab 2010;95(4):1708–16.

35. Gonzalez-Loyola A, Fernandez-Miranda G, Trakala M, et al. Aurora B overexpression causes aneuploidy and p21Cip1 repression during tumor development. Mol Cell Biol 2015;35(20):3566–78.

36. Tang A, Gao K, Chu L, et al. Aurora kinases: novel therapy targets in cancers. Oncotarget 2017;8(14): 23937–54.

37. Yuan J, Yan R, Kramer A, et al. Cyclin B1 depletion inhibits proliferation and induces apoptosis in human tumor cells. Oncogene 2004;23(34):5843–52.

38. Oh MC, Aghi MK. Dopamine agonist-resistant prolactinomas. J Neurosurg 2011;114(5):1369–79.

39. George DH, Scheithauer BW, Kovacs K, et al. Crooke's cell adenoma of the pituitary: an aggressive variant of corticotroph adenoma. Am J Surg Pathol 2003;27(10):1330–6.

40. Jahangiri A, Wagner JR, Pekmezci M, et al. A comprehensive long-term retrospective analysis of silent corticotrophic adenomas vs hormone-negative adenomas. Neurosurgery 2013;73(1):8–17 [discussion: 17–8].

41. Reincke M, Sbiera S, Hayakawa A, et al. Mutations in the deubiquitinase gene USP8 cause Cushing's disease. Nat Genet 2015;47(1):31–8.

42. Ma ZY, Song ZJ, Chen JH, et al. Recurrent gain-of-function USP8 mutations in Cushing's disease. Cell Res 2015;25(3):306–17.

43. Mizuno E, Iura T, Mukai A, et al. Regulation of epidermal growth factor receptor down-regulation by UBPY-mediated deubiquitination at endosomes. Mol Biol Cell 2005;16(11):5163–74.

44. Huang C, Shi Y, Zhao Y. USP8 mutation in Cushing's disease. Oncotarget 2015;6(21):18240–1.

45. Losa M, Mortini P, Pagnano A, et al. Clinical characteristics and surgical outcome in USP8-mutated human adrenocorticotropic hormone-secreting pituitary adenomas. Endocrine 2019; 63(2):240–6.

46. Song ZJ, Reitman ZJ, Ma ZY, et al. The genome-wide mutational landscape of pituitary adenomas. Cell Res 2016;26(11):1255–9.

47. Chen J, Jian X, Deng S, et al. Identification of recurrent USP48 and BRAF mutations in Cushing's disease. Nat Commun 2018;9(1):3171.

48. Salomon MP, Wang X, Marzese DM, et al. The epigenomic landscape of pituitary adenomas reveals specific alterations and differentiates among acromegaly, Cushing's disease and endocrine-inactive subtypes. Clin Cancer Res 2018;24(17): 4126–36.

49. Lu J, Chatain GP, Bugarini A, et al. Histone deacetylase inhibitor SAHA is a promising treatment of Cushing disease. J Clin Endocrinol Metab 2017; 102(8):2825–35.

50. Garbicz F, Mehlich D, Rak B, et al. Increased expression of the microRNA 106b~25 cluster and its host gene MCM7 in corticotroph pituitary adenomas is associated with tumor invasion and Crooke's cell morphology. Pituitary 2017;20(4): 450–63.

51. Zhou K, Zhang T, Fan Y, et al. MicroRNA-106b promotes pituitary tumor cell proliferation and invasion through PI3K/AKT signaling pathway by targeting PTEN. Tumour Biol 2016;37(10): 13469–77.

52. Du L, Bergsneider M, Mirsadraei L, et al. Evidence for orphan nuclear receptor TR4 in the etiology of Cushing disease. Proc Natl Acad Sci U S A 2013; 110(21):8555–60.

53. Riebold M, Kozany C, Freiburger L, et al. A C-terminal HSP90 inhibitor restores glucocorticoid sensitivity and relieves a mouse allograft model of Cushing disease. Nat Med 2015;21(3):276–80.

54. Chapman PB, Hauschild A, Robert C, et al. Improved survival with vemurafenib in melanoma with BRAF V600E mutation. N Engl J Med 2011; 364(26):2507–16.

55. Hauschild A, Grob JJ, Demidov LV, et al. Dabrafenib in BRAF-mutated metastatic melanoma: a multicentre, open-label, phase 3 randomised controlled trial. Lancet 2012;380(9839):358–65.

56. Brown NF, Carter T, Mulholland P. Dabrafenib in BRAFV600-mutated anaplastic pleomorphic xanthoastrocytoma. CNS Oncol 2017;6(1):5–9.

57. Cossu G, Daniel RT, Pierzchala K, et al. Thyrotropin-secreting pituitary adenomas: a systematic review and meta-analysis of postoperative outcomes and management. Pituitary 2019;22(1):79–88.

58. Beck-Peccoz P, Persani L, Lania A. Thyrotropin-secreting pituitary adenomas. In: De Groot LJ, Chrousos G, Dungan K, et al, editors. Endotext. South Dartmouth (MA): MDText.com, Inc; 2000.

59. Beck-Peccoz P, Persani L. Thyrotropinomas. Endocrinol Metab Clin North Am 2008;37(1):123–34. viii-ix.

60. Asteria C, Anagni M, Persani L, et al. Loss of heterozygosity of the MEN1 gene in a large series of TSH-secreting pituitary adenomas. J Endocrinol Invest 2001;24(10):796–801.

61. Sapkota S, Horiguchi K, Tosaka M, et al. Whole-exome sequencing study of thyrotropin-secreting pituitary adenomas. J Clin Endocrinol Metab 2017; 102(2):566–75.

62. Furumoto H, Ying H, Chandramouli GV, et al. An unliganded thyroid hormone beta receptor activates the cyclin D1/cyclin-dependent kinase/retinoblastoma/E2F pathway and induces pituitary tumorigenesis. Mol Cell Biol 2005;25(1):124–35.

63. Ando S, Sarlis NJ, Krishnan J, et al. Aberrant alternative splicing of thyroid hormone receptor in a TSH-secreting pituitary tumor is a mechanism for hormone resistance. Mol Endocrinol 2001;15(9): 1529–38.

64. Teng X, Jin T, Brent GA, et al. A patient with a thyrotropin-secreting microadenoma and resistance to thyroid hormone (P453T). J Clin Endocrinol Metab 2015;100(7):2511–4.

65. James RA, Sarapura VD, Bruns C, et al. Thyroid hormone-induced expression of specific somatostatin receptor subtypes correlates with involution of the TtT-97 murine thyrotrope tumor. Endocrinology 1997;138(2):719–24.

66. Yoshihara A, Isozaki O, Hizuka N, et al. Expression of type 5 somatostatin receptor in TSH-secreting pituitary adenomas: a possible marker for predicting long-term response to octreotide therapy. Endocr J 2007;54(1):133–8.

67. Wallace IR, Healy E, Cooke RS, et al. TSH-secreting pituitary adenoma: benefits of pre-operative octreotide. Endocrinol Diabetes Metab case Rep 2015; 2015:150007.

68. Fliers E, van Furth WR, Bisschop PH. Cure of a thyrotrophin (TSH)-secreting pituitary adenoma by medical therapy. Clin Endocrinol 2012;77(5):788–90.

69. Amlashi FG, Tritos NA. Thyrotropin-secreting pituitary adenomas: epidemiology, diagnosis, and management. Endocrine 2016;52(3):427–40.

70. Cote DJ, Smith TR, Sandler CN, et al. Functional gonadotroph adenomas: case series and report of literature. Neurosurgery 2016;79(6):823–31.

71. Newey PJ, Nesbit MA, Rimmer AJ, et al. Whole-exome sequencing studies of nonfunctioning

pituitary adenomas. J Clin Endocrinol Metab 2013; 98(4):E796–800.

72. Falch CM, Sundaram AYM, Oystese KA, et al. Gene expression profiling of fast- and slow-growing non-functioning gonadotroph pituitary adenomas. Eur J Endocrinol 2018;178(3):295–307.

73. Zhou Y, Zhong Y, Wang Y, et al. Activation of p53 by MEG3 non-coding RNA. J Biol Chem 2007;282(34): 24731–42.

74. Zhao J, Dahle D, Zhou Y, et al. Hypermethylation of the promoter region is associated with the loss of MEG3 gene expression in human pituitary tumors. J Clin Endocrinol Metab 2005;90(4):2179–86.

75. Chesnokova V, Zonis S, Wawrowsky K, et al. Clusterin and FOXL2 act concordantly to regulate pituitary gonadotroph adenoma growth. Mol Endocrinol 2012;26(12):2092–103.

76. Inoshita N, Nishioka H. The 2017 WHO classification of pituitary adenoma: overview and comments. Brain Tumor Pathol 2018;35(2):51–6.

77. Lee JC, Pekmezci M, Lavezo JL, et al. Utility of Pit-1 immunostaining in distinguishing pituitary adenomas of primitive differentiation from null cell adenomas. Endocr Pathol 2017;28(4):287–92.

78. Lin Y, Jiang X, Shen Y, et al. Frequent mutations and amplifications of the PIK3CA gene in pituitary tumors. Endocr Relat Cancer 2009;16(1):301–10.

79. Li H, Fredriksson L, Li X, et al. PDGF-D is a potent transforming and angiogenic growth factor. Oncogene 2003;22(10):1501–10.

80. Samuels Y, Diaz LA Jr, Schmidt-Kittler O, et al. Mutant PIK3CA promotes cell growth and invasion of human cancer cells. Cancer Cell 2005;7(6): 561–73.

81. Bahar A, Bicknell JE, Simpson DJ, et al. Loss of expression of the growth inhibitory gene GADD45gamma, in human pituitary adenomas, is associated with CpG island methylation. Oncogene 2004; 23(4):936–44.

82. Simpson DJ, Bicknell JE, McNicol AM, et al. Hypermethylation of the p16/CDKN2A/MTSI gene and loss of protein expression is associated with nonfunctional pituitary adenomas but not somatotrophinomas. Genes Chromosomes Cancer 1999;24(4): 328–36.

83. Butz H, Liko I, Czirjak S, et al. MicroRNA profile indicates downregulation of the TGFbeta pathway in sporadic non-functioning pituitary adenomas. Pituitary 2011;14(2):112–24.

Intraoperative Fluorescent Visualization of Pituitary Adenomas

Steve S. Cho, BS, John Y.K. Lee, MD, MSCE*

KEYWORDS

- Near-infrared fluorescence • Fluorescence-guided surgery • Second window indocyanine green
- SWIG • OTL38 • Pituitary adenomas

KEY POINTS

- Conventional endoscopic visualization with white light during pituitary adenomas resection often leads to incomplete resection due to inaccurate tissue identification.
- Near-infrared imaging has the potential to improve tumor detection capabilities in real time.
- Second window indocyanine green can be used in all pituitary adenomas regardless of secretory status and has superior sensitivity for neoplastic tissue compared with white light visualization alone.
- OTL38, which targets folate receptors, can be used in nonfunctional adenomas and has superior sensitivity and specificity for neoplastic tissue compared to white light alone.

INTRODUCTION

Complete resection of pituitary adenomas, which account for approximately 10% of intracranial tumors, can be curative; however, tumor recurrence rate can be as high as 20% after surgery due to incomplete resection and may require repeat surgery or other treatments.[1–6] The main factors that prevent a neurosurgeon from completely resecting pituitary adenomas are invasion of tumor into the cavernous sinus and involvement of the internal carotid artery, difficulty in distinguishing the adenoma from the normal pituitary stalk, and sometimes a lack of appreciation of where diaphragm sella starts/ends. Intraoperative neuronavigation is commonly used by neurosurgeons to localize intraparenchymal tumors as well as bony anatomy of the sinuses. Neuronavigation is fraught with errors, however, because the images for registration are obtained preoperatively and do not reflect anatomic changes in real time.[7] In addition, rapid changes in tumor position after debulking and diaphragm sella collapse can make interpretation of neuronavigation challenging. Intraoperative magnetic resonance imaging (MRI) may improve accuracy and resection rates but is associated with high cost and limited availability as well as high false-positive rates.[8,9] Thus, there remains a need for a simple, affordable, and rapid intraoperative imaging technique that offers real-time localization of neoplastic tissue. Recently, fluorescence-guided surgery (FGS) has emerged as a viable solution.

Disclosure Statement: S.S. Cho has nothing to disclose. J.Y.K. Lee owns stock options in Visionsense, which manufactures the endoscopes used for the research presented here. Supported in part by the National Institutes of Health R01 CA193556 (SS), and the Institute for Translational Medicine and Therapeutics of the Perelman School of Medicine at the University of Pennsylvania (JYKL). In addition, research reported in this publication was supported by the National Center for Advancing Translational Sciences of the National Institutes of Health under Award Number UL1TR000003 (JKYL). The content is solely the responsibility of the authors and does not necessarily represent the official views of the NIH.
Department of Neurosurgery, Perelman School of Medicine, University of Pennsylvania, Pennsylvania Hospital, 801 Spruce Street, 8th Floor, Philadelphia, PA, 19107, USA
* Corresponding author.
E-mail address: leejohn@uphs.upenn.edu

Currently, 5-aminolevulinic acid (ALA) remains the only Food and Drug Administration (FDA)-approved agent for tumor identification during surgery for suspected high-grade gliomas. It is a prodrug that has demonstrated sensitivity for neoplastic tissue and utility in increasing rates of gross total resection and improving progression-free survival in randomized control trials.[10–12] Some groups have attempted to investigate 5-ALA in pituitary adenomas resections.[13,14] Eljamel and colleagues[15] (30 patients with 14 nonfunctional adenomas) demonstrated that 80.8% of the adenomas demonstrated fluorescence after 5-ALA administration; no margin detection sensitivity and specificity were calculated in either study. Thus, the utility of 5-ALA in pituitary adenomas resection has not been investigated thoroughly and remains unclear.

In contrast to visible light fluorophores, the authors' research group has investigated the clinical utility of 2 near-infrared fluorescent dyes in pituitary adenoma resections.[16–18] In 2014, the authors initiated a study using delayed, high-dose imaging of indocyanine green (ICG). Second window ICG (SWIG) is an innovative application of a commonly used dye, ICG. This novel technique takes advantage of the enhanced vascular permeability of tumor tissue, allowing ICG to accumulate in peritumoral tissue over 24 hours (**Fig. 1**A). SWIG has been applied to real-time visualization of neoplastic tissue in gliomas, meningiomas, metastases, chordomas, craniopharyngiomas, and, finally, pituitary adenomas.[16,19–22] In 2015, the authors also began investigating the novel dye OTL38 (On Target Laboratories, West Lafayette, Indiana), which is a folate ligand linked to an ICG analog. OTL38 targets the folate receptor, which has been repeatedly demonstrated to be overexpressed in a large majority of nonfunctional pituitary adenomas (see **Fig. 1**B).[23–26] Both ICG and OTL38 emit fluorescence in the near-infrared region (700–850 nm), which confers 2 main advantages over visible-light spectrum fluorophores, such as 5-ALA or fluorescein: increased tissue penetration by the photons (>10 mm through brain and dura vs <1 mm for visible light) and significantly lower background signal from brain autofluorescence.[27,28]

This report describes the technique for intraoperative fluorescent visualization of pituitary adenomas using SWIG and OTL38 and summarizes the main outcomes of the authors' prior studies.

INDICATIONS/CONTRAINDICATIONS

ICG is the only FDA-approved near-infrared fluorophore for use in human patients. Its low toxicity and good safety profile allow it to be used in most patients with intracranial tumors. The main indication for the use of SWIG is a radiographic diagnosis of an intracranial tumor in a patient over the age of 18 years. Although the authors have demonstrated previously that contrast enhancement with gadolinium positively correlates with intraoperative near-infrared fluorescence signal with SWIG, contrast enhancement is not a prerequisite. The major contraindication for SWIG is allergy to iodide, contrast dye, or shellfish, because some preparations of ICG contain sodium iodide. Anaphylactic reactions and other severe adverse reactions are rare (<0.1%).[29]

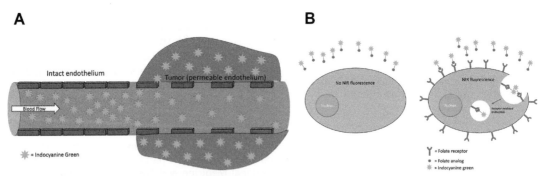

Fig. 1. Mechanism of action for SWIG and OTL38. ICG is hypothesized to accumulate in tumor tissues via the enhanced permeability and retention effect (*A*). Benign tissue with intact endothelium is minimally permeable to small molecules, but tumor tissue with damaged and/or disrupted vasculature allows these small molecules to diffuse into and be retained within the tissue. In the case of SWIG, the ideal time frame is approximately 24 hours for this accumulation to have increased specificity for tumor tissue. Receptor-targeting dyes (*B*), on the other hand, bind specifically to cells that express the target receptors (*Right*), whereas cells that do not express the receptors (*Left*) do not accumulate the dye. OTL38 binds to and is internalized by folate receptors, which are overexpressed on nonfunctional pituitary adenomas. NIR, near-infrared. (*From* Cho SS, Jeon J, Buch L, et al. Intraoperative near-infrared imaging with receptor-specific versus passive delivery of fluorescent agents in pituitary adenomas. J Neurosurg. 2018;14:1–11; with permission.)

Another contraindication to SWIG is pregnancy, because the safety profiles of receiving ICG in the significantly higher dose required for SWIG has not been investigated in pregnant women.

With OTL38, its safety profile remains reasonable, because it is composed of a folate analog linked to an ICG analog, both of which have low toxicities. The primary indication for the use of OTL38 currently is a radiographic diagnosis of a pituitary adenoma in a patient over the age of 18 years, with serum hormone levels suggesting that the adenoma is a nonfunctional adenoma. An additional exclusion criterion beyond those of SWIG is allergy to folate-containing supplements, because OTL38 contains a folate analog.

The inclusion and exclusion criteria for SWIG and OTL38 are listed in **Table 1**.

SURGICAL TECHNIQUE/PROCEDURE
Preoperative Planning

ICG for SWIG and OTL38 must be administered intravenously to patients 24 hours and 3 hours preoperatively, respectively. This may be done at an outpatient infusion suite for ICG or in the preoperative patient holding area the day of surgery for OTL38. ICG is administered at a dose of 5 mg/kg of bodyweight, whereas OTL38 is administered at 0.025 mg/kg of bodyweight. Both drugs are infused over 45 minutes to 60 minutes; if a patient develops discomfort and/or itchiness, the infusion can be slowed down to more than 90 minutes. Patients receiving OTL38 should be instructed to discontinue all folate-containing supplements and vitamins for 3 days to 4 days prior to surgery, to minimize interactions with OTL38.

Table 1
Indications and contraindications for fluorescence-guided surgery with near-infrared fluorophores

Fluorescent Dye Agent	Indications	Contraindications
SWIG	Diagnosis of intracranial tumor	Allergy to iodide, contrast dye, or shellfish
	Age >18 y	Pregnancy
OTL38	Diagnosis of pituitary adenomas	Allergy to iodide, contrast dye, or shellfish
	Age >18 y	Pregnancy
	Serum testing suggesting nonsecretory adenoma	Allergy to folate-containing supplements

Preparation and Patient Positioning/Surgical Approach

The use of SWIG or OTL38 does not alter the patient positioning, prepping, or surgical approach.

Equipment

To visualize near-infrared fluorescence, a dedicated white light and near-infrared light endoscope is needed. There are multiple options in the market, but the Visionsense Iridium system (Visionsense, Philadelphia, PA, USA) has been shown in prior studies to have superb near-infrared sensitivity and dynamic range.[30,31] For ICG, this system uses an 805-nm laser to excite ICG at its peak excitation and records emission at wavelengths 820 nm to 860 nm; for OTL38, the laser is tuned to 785 nm and emissions between 800 nm and 835 nm are recorded (**Fig. 2**). The endoscope version of the Visionsense Iridium offers video imaging at 1080 pixels (recording saved at 720cpixels) through a 0°, 4-mm outer diameter scope. No angled scopes are currently available. Due to the lack of angled scopes and lower resolution than the high-definition endoscopes, a surgeon may choose to use the usual endoscope for the majority of the case, using the Visionsense Iridium only when necessary to image in the near-infrared (**Fig. 3**).

Visualization Technique

Near-infrared visualization with an endoscope presents a unique challenge that imaging with exoscopes or microscopes does not. Because light decays exponentially as a factor of distance squared, having the scope twice as close results in fluorescence signal that is 16-times higher (4-times stronger excitation light and 4-times more emission reaching the sensor). Thus, bringing the scope too proximal to any tissue can result in artificially elevated near-infrared fluorescence measurement simply by flooding the area with excitation photons. This is further complicated with endoscopes because the narrow diameter of the scope requires a pinpoint excitation light source. This focal excitation light results in more excitation light in the center of the field and less at the periphery, causing vignetting with kurtosis toward the center of the view (**Fig. 4**). Thus, tissue in the center of the viewing area may appear to fluoresce relative to the surrounding background simply due to this vignetting, resulting in false-positive fluorescence measurement. In a prior publication, the authors quantified and standardized the optimal distance for pituitary adenoma resections using the Visionsense Iridium endoscope. Using intraoperative landmarks, the authors chose the bilateral medial opticocarotid

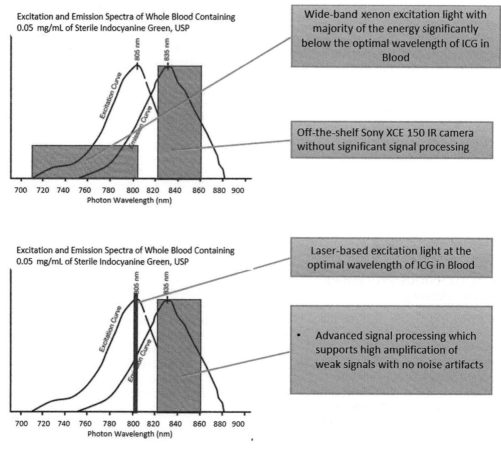

Fig. 2. Near-infrared visualization. The Visionsense Iridium system is the leading product in the market for both exoscope and endoscope visualization of near-infrared fluorophores intraoperatively. Unlike conventional surgical microscopes or modified endoscopes, which often use a broadband xenon light to excite the near-infrared fluorophore (*above*), the Visionsense uses a tuned laser that delivers the maximum number of photons at the peak excitation wavelength (*below*). This, combined with sophisticated image processing, gives the Visionsense unrivalled sensitivity and dynamic range for intraoperative near-infrared visualization. (*Adapted from* Cho SS, Zeh R, Pierce JT, et al. Comparison of near-infrared imaging camera systems for intracranial tumor detection. Mol Imaging Biol. 2018;20(2):213–220; with permission.)

recess (MOCR) as an internal reference point, because the MOCR has been previously demonstrated to be a reliable anatomic landmark (see **Fig. 3I**).[32–34] In the authors' studies with OTL38, adenomas that did not overexpress folate receptors only fluoresced when the scope was in close proximity to the tumor (ie, MOCR >50% of the screen), whereas adenomas with folate receptor overexpression fluoresced strongly regardless of the scope distance (**Fig. 5**). Thus, the authors demonstrated that obtaining near-infrared imaging while maintaining the distance between the bilateral MOCR to be less than 50% of the overall visual field offered the best discrimination between truly fluorescent areas and false-positive areas. Thus, neurosurgeons should be aware of maintaining proper distance when measuring near-infrared fluorescence, while understanding that different

endoscopes may have different vignetting profiles or may offer more exact distance measurements.

Surgical Procedure

- Step 1: after standard patient position and prepping, an uninostril or binostril endoscopic endonasal approach is performed. The choice of approach is made based on patient anatomy.
- Step 2: open both sphenoid sinuses, remove the sphenoid rostrum, and resect the sphenoid intersinus septum.
- Step 3: remove the mucosa of the sella and obtain hemostasis to minimize blood contamination of the field.
- Step 4: after exposing the sella face and floor, open the sella using standard techniques.

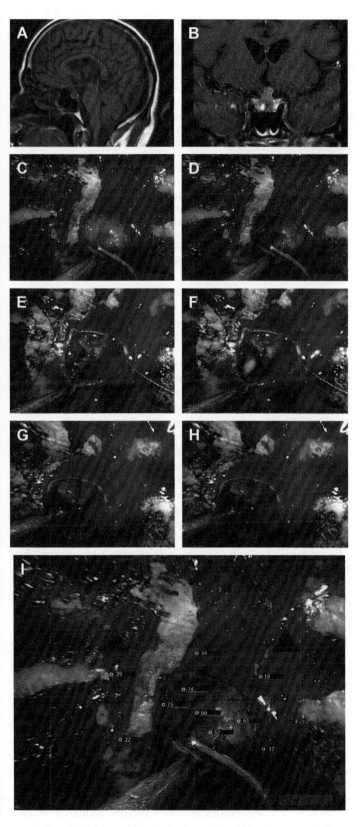

Fig. 3. Intraoperative endoscopic near-infrared imaging techniques. A patient presented with a 17-mm nonfunctional macroadenoma with folate receptor overexpression (*A, B*). The Visionsense endoscope simultaneously displays the white light view (*C, E, G*) and the near-infrared view (*D, F, H*) in real-time overlay, which can help surgeons maintain context of the surrounding area while visualizing fluorescent areas. The tumor was visible once the dura is opened (*C, D*). After resection (*E, F*), residual fluorescent tissue was visualized, which was removed; on pathology, this specimen was neoplastic. Postresection view (*G, H*) demonstrates no residual fluorescence. Demonstrated (*I*) are the 2 MOCRs (*black triangles*), which span approximately 50% of the surgical view, which the authors used as a surrogate to measure distance from the tissue to maintain optimal distance for near-infrared imaging. Five points of interests (*white circles*) were each chosen at random on the tumor and on the surrounding tissue to calculate the SBR for the near-infrared fluorescence (2.8 in this case). (*From* Lee JYK, Cho SS, Zeh R, et al. Folate receptor overexpression can be visualized in real time during pituitary adenoma endoscopic transsphenoidal surgery with near-infrared imaging. J Neurosurg. 2018;129(2):390–403; with permission.)

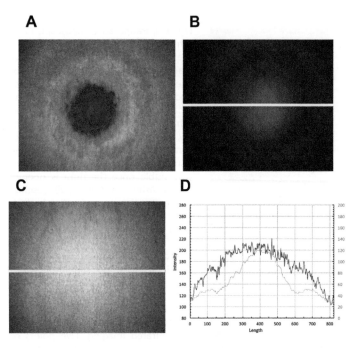

A

B

C

D

Fig. 4. Vignetting of illumination light with endoscopes. In this demonstration, the Visionsense endoscope was used to visualize a uniformly ICG-enriched control. As seen in the overlay (*A*) and near-infrared–only (*B*) views, the center of the field has more signal although the signal should be uniform across the visualization field. Using the signal intensity along the middle of the field (*B, C* [*yellow lines*]), the near-infrared laser vignetting (*D* [*light blue line*]) is more severe than the white light (*D* [*black line*]) (kurtosis 1.96 vs 2.40). (*From* Jeon J, Cho SS, Nag S, et al. Near-infrared optical contrast of skull base tumors during endoscopic endonasal surgery. Oper Neurosurg. 2018; with permission.)

- Step 5: once the dura surrounding the sella turcica is revealed, use the Visionsense scope to locate the tumor through the dura.
- Step 6: after confirming tumor location, incise the dura to expose the underlying tumor and possibly normal pituitary gland.
- Step 7: use the Visionsense scope to establish baseline near-infrared fluorescence signal prior to resection. This helps establish the degree of fluorescence in preparation for margin detection.
- Step 8: resect the tumor under white light using standard-of-care techniques, while using near-infrared imaging intermittently to establish margins. The authors' unpublished data (John Y. K. Lee, personal communication) suggest that the pars nervosa (posterior neurohypophysis) can be brightly fluorescent, so beware of chasing high signal. Normal pituitary gland and dura do not tend to be very bright with SWIG or OTL38.
- Step 9: after satisfactory resection, perform near-infrared imaging of the resection bed. If there are remnant areas of fluorescence, the surgeon should make an informed decision as to whether to further resect or not.
- Step 10: closure in the standard-of-care manner. Use free mucosal graft or nasoseptal flap as necessary for secure closure.

COMPLICATIONS AND MANAGEMENT

To date, no significant adverse events have been associated with the use of either SWIG or OTL38

in patients. In less than 5% of cases, patients may report mild to moderate pruritus at the infusion site or distal sites and/or moderate pain at the intravenous site during the infusion; the authors have found that administering diphenhydramine relieves the pruritus, whereas applying a heat pad and decreasing the rate of infusion resolve the pain.

No surgical complications related to intravenous dye infusion have been identified in the authors' cohort of patients. The rates of postoperative diabetes insipidus, syndrome of inappropriate antidiuretic hormone, or visual field deficits have not been significantly different from those of prior cohorts of patients. It is important to acknowledge that in the authors' studies, the extent of resection was not changed significantly based on the near-infrared imaging. In essence, if a surgeon would not have resected the tissue otherwise, he/she did not resect the areas of residual fluorescence. Biopsies have been taken, however, when appropriate to measure sensitivity/specificity of the dye as a diagnostic test.

POSTOPERATIVE CARE

Unlike with 5-ALA, which requires patients to be protected from the sun and other ultraviolet radiation for 24 hours after surgery, the use of SWIG and OTL38 does not preclude discharge from the hospital or limit patient activity if safe to do so otherwise. Patients' sodium levels and urine output should be monitored per standard protocol. Routine follow-up care should be performed according to institutional protocols.

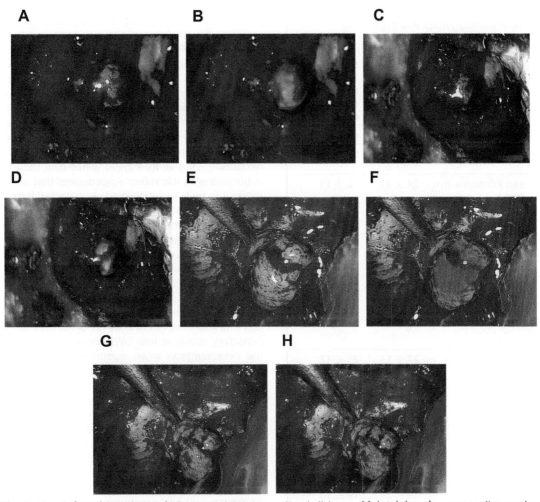

Fig. 5. Near-infrared imaging technique—maintaining optimal distance. Maintaining the proper distance between the near-infrared camera and the tissue of interest is crucial in obtaining accurate near-infrared signal without high false-positive rates. Because near-infrared signal increases as a factor of distance to the fourth power, being close to the tissue can cause excessive excitation leading to false-positive signal. Truly fluorescent tumors and tissue should fluoresce strongly regardless of the distance between the scope and the tissue. In a patient with a nonfunctional adenoma with very high expression of folate receptors, the adenoma fluoresces with an SBR of 3.9 when the MOCR spans 75% of the field (*A, B*). The SBR remains high, at 3.3, when the scope is moved further away and the MOCR spans 30% of the field (*C, D*). Conversely, an adenoma with almost no folate receptor expression fluoresces with an SBR of 2.1 when the MOCR spans 70% of the field (*E, F*), but the SBR decreases significantly to 1.1 when the scope is moved further away (*G, H*). (*Adapted from* Lee JYK, Cho SS, Zeh R, et al. Folate receptor overexpression can be visualized in real time during pituitary adenoma endoscopic transsphenoidal surgery with near-infrared imaging. J Neurosurg. 2018;129(2):390–403; with permission.)

OUTCOMES

To date, 39 patients with pituitary adenomas (23 OTL38 and 16 SWIG) have undergone transsphenoidal endoscopic resection with near-infrared imaging. Detailed demographic and clinical information is summarized in **Table 2**.[16] Although the extent of resection was not modified in these studies, margin specimens were biopsied during the case and each specimen was observed under white light alone and under near-infrared imaging. Using histopathology as the gold standard of tissue identity, the accuracy of each technique was calculated, as discussed later.

With SWIG, both hormone-secreting and nonsecreting adenomas demonstrated strong near-infrared fluorescence intraoperatively with average signal-to-background ratio (SBR) of 4.1 ± 0.72. Of a total of 30 specimens in 16 patients, SWIG was

Table 2
Patient demographics and presenting symptoms in each study group

	OTL38 (23 Cases)	Second Window Indocyanine Green (16 Cases)
Male (%)	52	56
Mean age (y)	54.0 ± 17.5	57.4 ± 11.0
Mean adenoma size (mm)	24 ± 13	22 ± 11
Prior pituitary surgery (%)	17.4	18.8
Prior pituitary radiation (%)	0	0
Mean time from contrast agent infusion to visualization (h)	4.8 ± 1.2	22 ± 2.4
Nonfunctioning adenoma (n)	14	7
Mean adenoma size (mm)	27 ± 13	25 ± 12
Macroadenoma (n)	14	7
Visual field compromise (n)	6	2
Cavernous sinus invasion (n)	12	7
Functioning adenoma (n)	9	9
Mean adenoma size (mm)	18 ± 11	19 ± 10
Macroadenoma (n)	8	7
Cushing disease (n)	6	2
Acromegaly (n)	3	4
Prolactinoma (n)	0	2
Thyrotroph adenoma (n)	0	1

Data are numbers of cases unless otherwise indicated. Mean values are presented with SDs.

From Cho SS, Jeon J, Buch L, et al. Intraoperative near-infrared imaging with receptor-specific versus passive delivery of fluorescent agents in pituitary adenomas. J Neurosurg. 2018;14:1–11; with permission.

100% sensitive and 29% specific, with 82% positive-predictive value (PPV) and 100% negative-predictive value (NPV) for neoplastic tissue. With white light visualization alone, the neurosurgeon demonstrated 88% sensitivity, 90% specificity, 96% PPV, and 73% NPV. Thus, consistent with the authors' results in other intracranial tumors, near-infrared imaging with SWIG was more sensitive for neoplastic tissue, with a higher NPV, but was less specific and thus suffered in its PPV. This is because SWIG is not a tumor-specific technique; rather, it accumulates in stroma with disrupted endothelium and poor capillary clearance, which also can occur in areas of inflammation or necrosis. In the authors' studies, near-infrared imaging with SWIG in pituitary adenomas had 0 false-negative results; if the tissue was not fluorescent, it was always non-neoplastic. On the other hand, white light visualization alone misclassified 7 specimens that were thought to be non-neoplastic but contained tumor tissue on pathology. Thus, near-infrared imaging with SWIG can help the neurosurgeon avoid resecting normal tissue in cases where tissue identity is not certain. If the tissue in question does not fluoresce with SWIG, it significantly increases the likelihood that it is not neoplastic and thus should not be resected. Overall, if the goal of the surgery is to achieve total resection and leave as little tumor behind as possible, the higher sensitivity achieved with SWIG could greatly help the neurosurgeon when combined with careful judgment to prevent resecting normal tissue.

In this published pilot study, OTL38 was administered to all patients with pituitary adenomas, regardless of functional status. It was soon recognized, however, that functional adenomas did not overexpress folate receptors and thus had very low near-infrared fluorescence (average SBR 1.7 ± 0.47). Postoperative immunohistochemistry confirmed that none of the functional adenomas overexpressed folate receptor alpha, which is the target binding site for OTL38. This was consistent with prior studies looking at folate receptor expression.[23–26] In contrast, nonfunctional adenomas demonstrated significantly stronger fluorescence (SBR = 2.6 ± 0.91) and folate receptor overexpression was seen in 64% (9/14) of cases, again consistent with prior studies. In nonfunctional adenomas, OTL38 demonstrated 75% sensitivity, 100% specificity, 100% PPV, and 62% NPV; in the 9 adenomas that overexpressed folate receptors, near-infrared fluorescence was even stronger (SBR = 3.2 ± 0.53) and sensitivity, specificity, PPV, and NPV were all 100%. In comparison, white light alone demonstrated 83% sensitivity, 100% specificity, 100% PPV, and 89% NPV. One caveat, however, is that folate receptor expression levels cannot easily be determined preoperatively. Thus, the authors concluded that all patients with nonfunctional adenomas should be considered for near-infrared FGS with OTL38, but if there is no significant fluorescence on exposing the tumor, it should be assumed that the tumor does not overexpress folate receptors and the rest of the surgery should proceed without near-infrared imaging.

Another method of validating the authors' imaging technique was to correlate intraoperative molecular imaging with postoperative MRI scans. Although the authors did not alter the extent of resection based on near-infrared fluorescence imaging, they compared residual near-infrared fluorescence using either fluorophore with postoperative MRI. Near-infrared imaging with SWIG was able to predict postoperative MRI results in 9 of 12 patients, with 1 false-negative result and 2 false-positive results. Near-infrared imaging with OTL38 was able to predict postoperative MRI results in 8 of 9 patients with folate receptor overexpressing adenomas, with 1 false-negative result. An example of prediction of residual neoplasm is shown in **Fig. 6**. The false-negative results

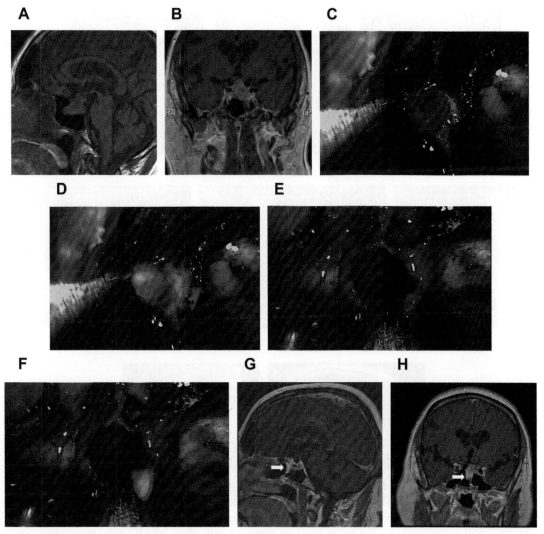

Fig. 6. Prediction of postoperative MRI with near-infrared imaging. Patient presented with a 27-mm, Knosp grade 2 nonfunctional adenoma (*A, B*). Tumor could be visualized with white light (*C*) and near-infrared (*D*) on opening the dura. After standard resection, no obvious residual neoplasm was appreciated with white light (*E*), but near-infrared imaging demonstrated strongly fluorescent residual area (*F*), which was not biopsied. Postoperative MRI demonstrating residual tumor in the anterior sella region (*white arrow*), consistent with the fluorescent area seen in (*G, H*). (*From* Cho SS, Zeh R, Pierce JT, et al. Folate receptor near-infrared optical imaging provides sensitive and specific intraoperative visualization of nonfunctional pituitary adenomas. Oper Neurosurg. 2019;16(1):59–70; with permission.)

were thought to due to the lack of angled endoscopes in the Visionsense system, which precluded the neurosurgeon from being able visualize tissue (especially around the cavernous sinus and frontal lobe tumor) that may have been fluorescent if it were in direct line of sight of the endoscope (**Fig. 7**). Overall, with both SWIG and OTL38, the absence of near-infrared fluorescence after surgical resection strongly correlated with total resection of the adenoma on postoperative MRI, suggesting that resecting all fluorescent tissue may increase the likelihood of achieving total resection. Based on these findings, the authors think that near-infrared imaging can predict MRI results, especially if angled, near-infrared capable endoscopes were available.

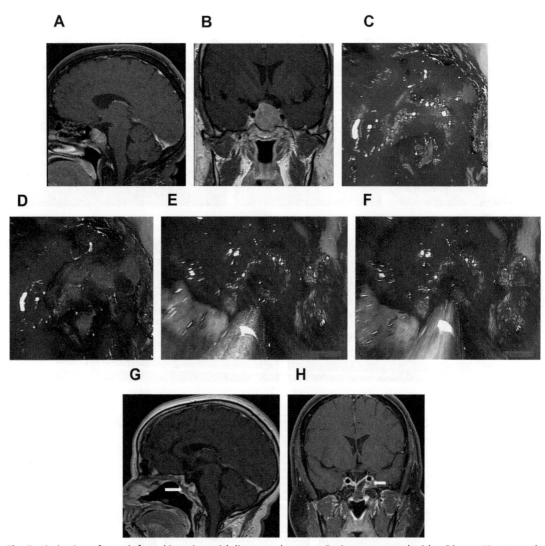

Fig. 7. Limitation of near-infrared imaging with linear endoscopes. Patient presented with a 20-mm, Knosp grade 4 nonfunctional adenoma (*A*, *B*). The tumor could be visualized with white light (*C*) and near-infrared (*D*) on opening the dura. After standard resection, no obvious residual neoplasm was appreciated with white light (*E*), but an area of residual fluorescence was visualized in the center of the surgical field (*F*), which was not biopsied. On postoperative MRI, an area of residual neoplasm was visualized (*G* [*arrow*]). The residual neoplasm around the left cavernous sinus (*H* [*arrow*]), however, had not been visualized in (*F*). Thus, a major limitation of the previous studies is the lack of angled endoscopes, which likely limited the visualization of residual fluorescence around corners into the cavernous sinus. (*From* Cho SS, Zeh R, Pierce JT, et al. Folate receptor near-infrared optical imaging provides sensitive and specific intraoperative visualization of nonfunctional pituitary adenomas. Oper Neurosurg. 2019;16(1):59–70; with permission.)

SUMMARY

Surgical resection for pituitary adenomas remains the primary form of treatment, often occurring prior to radiation or chemotherapy or when pharmacologic therapy has failed. Incomplete resection, however, resulting in tumor recurrence is common. Fluorescence-guided tumor surgery is a developing technique that may help neurosurgeons achieve more accurate distinction between tumor and the surrounding tissue to achieve maximal safe resection of intracranial tumors. This article summarizes the authors' experience with SWIG, a novel technique that relies on the passive accumulation of ICG in tumors via the enhanced permeability and retention effect and is broadly applicable to all pituitary adenomas regardless of functional status. OTL38 is an investigational near-infrared dye that targets folate receptors on nonfunctional adenomas with exquisite sensitivity and specificity for neoplastic tissue. Both techniques work in the near-infrared region, allowing the surgeon to visualize fluorescent tissue that may be hidden behind normal tissue with strong contrast against the normal background. The authors' efforts represent the first step in near-infrared fluorescence guided surgery of pituitary adenomas and should encourage other neurosurgeons to consider these techniques as well as other novel dyes to improve surgical outcomes.

REFERENCES

1. Ezzat S, Asa SL, Couldwell WT, et al. The prevalence of pituitary adenomas. Cancer 2004;101:613–9.

2. Greenman Y, Cooper O, Yaish I, et al. Treatment of clinically nonfunctioning pituitary adenomas with dopamine agonists. Eur J Endocrinol 2016;175: 63–72.

3. Lee JYK, Bohman L-E, Bergsneider M. Contemporary neurosurgical techniques for pituitary tumor resection. J Neurooncol 2014;117:437–44.

4. Losa M, Mortini P, Barzaghi R, et al. Early results of surgery in patients with nonfunctioning pituitary adenoma and analysis of the risk of tumor recurrence. J Neurosurg 2008;108:525–32.

5. Thawani JP, Ramayya AG, Pisapia JM, et al. Operative strategies to minimize complications following resection of pituitary macroadenomas. J Neurol Surg B Skull Base 2017;78:184–90.

6. Sheehan J, Lee CC, Bodach ME, et al. Congress of neurological surgeons systematic review and evidence-based guideline for the management of patients with residual or recurrent nonfunctioning pituitary adenomas. Neurosugery 2016;79:E539–40.

7. Corlu A, Choe R, Durduran T, et al. Chapter functional imaging with diffusing light. Optics express. In: Yodh, Boas DA, editors. Biomedical photonics, vol. 48. CRC Press; 1995. p. 1128–39.

8. Berkmann S, Schlaffer S, Nimsky C, et al. Follow-up and long-term outcome of nonfunctioning pituitary adenoma operated by transsphenoidal surgery with intraoperative high-field magnetic resonance imaging. Acta Neurochir (Wien) 2014. https://doi.org/10.1007/s00701-014-2210-x

9. Berkmann S, Schlaffer S, Nimsky C, et al. Intraoperative high-field MRI for transsphenoidal reoperations of nonfunctioning pituitary adenoma. J Neurosurg 2014;121:1–10.

10. Stummer W, Pichlmeier U, Meinel T, et al, ALA-Glioma Study Group. Fluorescence-guided surgery with 5-aminolevulinic acid for resection of malignant glioma: a randomised controlled multicentre phase III trial. Lancet Oncol 2006;7: 392–401.

11. Piquer Belloch J, Rovira V, Llácer JL, et al. Fluorescence-guided surgery in high grade gliomas using an exoscope system. Acta Neurochir (Wien) 2014; 156:653–60.

12. Stummer W, Novotny A, Stepp H, et al. Fluorescence-guided resection of glioblastoma multiforme by using 5-aminolevulinic acid-induced porphyrins: a prospective study in 52 consecutive patients. J Neurosurg 2000;93:1003–13.

13. Sam M, Ae E, Ae GL, et al. Intraoperative optical identification of pituitary adenomas. J Neurooncol 2009;92:417–21.

14. Marbacher S, Klinger E, Schwyzer L, et al. Use of fluorescence to guide resection or biopsy of primary brain tumors and brain metastases. Neurosurg Focus 2014;36:E10.

15. Eljamel MS, Leese G, Moseley H. Intraoperative optical identification of pituitary adenomas. J Neurooncol 2009;92:417–21.

16. Cho SS, Jeon J, Buch L, et al. Intraoperative near-infrared imaging with receptor-specific versus passive delivery of fluorescent agents in pituitary adenomas. J Neurosurg 2018;1:1–11.

17. Lee JYK, Cho SS, Zeh R, et al. Folate receptor overexpression can be visualized in real time during pituitary adenoma endoscopic transsphenoidal surgery with near-infrared imaging. J Neurosurg 2018. https://doi.org/10.3171/2017.2.JNS163191.

18. Cho SS, Zeh R, Pierce JT, et al. Folate receptor near-infrared optical imaging provides sensitive and specific intraoperative visualization of nonfunctional pituitary adenomas. Oper Neurosurg (Hagerstown) 2018. https://doi.org/10.1093/ons/opy034.

19. Jeon JW, Cho SS, Nag S, et al. Near-infrared optical contrast of skull base tumors during endoscopic endonasal surgery. Oper Neurosurg (Hagerstown) 2019;17(1):32–42.

20. Lee JYK, Thawani JP, Pierce J, et al. Intraoperative near-infrared optical imaging can localize gadolinium-enhancing gliomas during surgery. Neurosurgery 2016;79:856–71.

21. Lee JYK, Pierce JT, Zeh R, et al. Intraoperative near-infrared optical contrast can localize brain metastases. World Neurosurg 2017;106:120–30.

22. Lee JYK, Pierce JT, Thawani JP, et al. Near-infrared fluorescent image-guided surgery for intracranial meningioma. J Neurosurg 2018;128:380–90.

23. Galt JR, Halkar RK, Evans CO, et al. In vivo assay of folate receptors in nonfunctional pituitary adenomas with 99m Tc-Folate SPECT/CT. J Nucl Med 2010;51: 1716–23.

24. Evans C-O, Reddy P, Brat DJ, et al. Differential expression of folate receptor in pituitary adenomas. Cancer Res 2003;63:4218–24.

25. Evans C-O, Yao C, Laborde D, et al. Folate receptor expression in pituitary adenomas cellular and molecular analysis. Vitam Horm 2008;79:235–66.

26. Evans C-O, Young AN, Brown MR, et al. Novel patterns of gene expression in pituitary adenomas identified by complementary deoxyribonucleic acid microarrays and quantitative reverse transcription-polymerase chain reaction. J Clin Endocrinol Metab 2001;86:3097–107.

27. Frangioni JV. In vivo near-infrared fluorescence imaging. Curr Opin Chem Biol 2003;7:626–34.

28. Padalkar MV, Pleshko N. Wavelength-dependent penetration depth of near infrared radiation into cartilage. Analyst 2015;140:2093–100.

29. Hope-Ross M, Yannuzzi LA, Gragoudas ES, et al. Adverse reactions due to indocyanine green. Ophthalmology 1994;101:529–33.

30. Dsouza AV, Lin H, Henderson ER, et al. Review of fluorescence guided surgery systems: identification of key performance capabilities beyond indocyanine green imaging. J Biomed Opt 2016. https://doi.org/10.1117/1.JBO.21.8.080901.

31. Cho SS, Zeh R, Pierce JT, et al. Comparison of near-infrared imaging camera systems for intracranial tumor detection. Mol Imaging Biol 2018;20: 213–20.

32. Kikuchi R, Toda M, Wakahara S, et al. Analysis of the medial opticocarotid recess in patients with pituitary macroadenoma using three-dimensional images. World Neurosurg 2016;93: 139–43.

33. Labib MA, Prevedello DM, Fernandez-Miranda JC, et al. The medial opticocarotid recess: an anatomic study of an endoscopic "key landmark" for the ventral cranial base. Neurosurgery 2013;72(1 Suppl Operative):66–76.

34. Yang Y, Zhan G, Liao J, et al. Morphological characteristics of the sphenoid sinus and endoscopic localization of the cavernous sinus. J Craniofac Surg 2015;26:1983–7.

Intraoperative MRI for Pituitary Adenomas

Pamela S. Jones, MD, MS, MPH[a],*, Brooke Swearingen, MD[b]

KEYWORDS

- Intraoperative MRI • Pituitary tumor • Pituitary macroadenomas • Optic chiasm compression

KEY POINTS

- Goals of surgical management of pituitary adenomas are maximal safe resection, maintenance/restoration of abnormal hormone function, and functional restoration of neurologic deficits attributed to mass effect.
- Use of intraoperative MRI (iMRI) can provide real-time assessment that is both sensitive and specific for residual tumor.
- iMRI can increase the likelihood of achieving a gross total resection by up to 40%.
- iMRI finding of optic apparatus decompression is predictive of visual recovery in most patients.

INTRODUCTION

Surgery has been the mainstay of treatment for pituitary adenomas over the last 120 years. Largely performed via the transsphenoidal route pioneered by Harvey Cushing and Oskar Hirsch, this neurosurgical procedure carries an overall low mortality and morbidity rate.[1] Surgical excision is the treatment of choice for most pituitary tumors that secrete hormones, except for prolactinomas, whereby surgery is reserved for cases of medication resistance or intolerance. Surgery for nonfunctioning tumors is typically recommended when tumors are larger than 1 cm (macroadenomas), are growing, are causing pituitary insufficiency, or are compromising vision because of pressure on the optic apparatus. The goals of surgery are maximal safe resection and restoration of neurologic deficits attributed to mass effect, and, in functioning tumors, normalization of endocrinopathies. Long-term outcomes for these tumors are favorable, with low rates of recurrence, especially when GTR of tumor is achieved.[2] However, medical management following surgery may be required for biochemical control of acromegaly and Cushing disease, and radiation treatment of tumors may also be necessary for growth control and/or biochemical remission.

Since the 1990s, MRI scanners have been incorporated into the operating room environment and can provide near–real-time MRI for both intraoperative orientation and determination of the adequacy of resection. Studies of the use of intraoperative MRI (iMRI) for pituitary adenomas have shown that images are sensitive and specific for residual tumor detection. Furthermore, imaging allows for real-time assessment of residual tumor in surgically accessible versus nonaccessible areas and, thus, has been found to increase the likelihood of gross total resection (GTR). Owing to the slow-growing nature of pituitary adenomas, comparison of long-term control rates with and without use of iMRI remains to be studied, but the increased rates of GTR with this technology promise that this will lead to improved long-term outcomes.

HISTORY OF INTRAOPERATIVE MRI

The origin of iMRI for neurosurgery began at Brigham and Women's Hospital at Harvard Medical

Disclosure Statement: The authors have nothing to disclose.
[a] Department of Neurosurgery, Massachusetts General Hospital, Harvard Medical School, 15 Parkman Street, WAC 745, Boston, MA 02114, USA; [b] Department of Neurosurgery, Massachusetts General Hospital, Harvard Medical School, 15 Parkman Street, WAC 3, Boston, MA 02114, USA
* Corresponding author.
E-mail address: psjones@partners.org

Neurosurg Clin N Am 30 (2019) 413–420
https://doi.org/10.1016/j.nec.2019.05.003
1042-3680/19/© 2019 Elsevier Inc. All rights reserved.

School in the 1980 and 1990s in a collaborative effort between the departments of radiology, neurosurgery, otolaryngology, and General Electric Medical Systems. They developed an open-configuration MRI scanner of "double-doughnut" magnets that allowed surgery to be performed with concurrent intraoperative image guidance between the 2 magnets.[3] Although the advantages of this system were that the patient did not have to be moved and it allowed for real-time stereotaxy, the image resolution from magnet strength of the 0.5-T field was poor in comparison with diagnostic 1.5-T and 3-T MRI scanners.

Several other iMRI systems have been introduced since the 1990s, including the IMRIS system (Deerfield Imaging, Minnetonka, MN), a rail-mounted MRI that also allows for minimal movement of the patient. At the Massachusetts General Hospital, we have used a 3T IMRIS system for all of our iMRI cases since 2012. IMRIS was developed by a Canadian neurosurgeon, Garnette Sutherland, and launched commercially in 2005. The 70-cm bore, 1.5-T or 3-T scanner is stored in a magnet room between 2 operating rooms, and via a ceiling-mounted rail system the magnet is able to move into each operating room (Fig. 1). The operating suite is designed around the IMRIS magnet, stored behind radiofrequency-shielded and sound-shielded doors, and includes an MR-compatible operating room table and head fixation devices specifically designed to fit with the IMRIS operating room table and the IMRIS radiofrequency coils. To date, more than 60 IMRIS systems have been installed worldwide, with thousands of surgeries performed.

Other systems include portable MRI units, such as the Medtronic PoleStar (Medtronic, Minneapolis, MN), which allows iMRI to be performed without significant modifications made to the operating room suite. However, these are low-field units, and reports are mixed on the effects on rates of resection with this imaging.

INTRAOPERATIVE MRI FOR PITUITARY TUMOR RESECTION

The real-world value of iMRI systems is in detecting actionable unexpected tumor residuals. Currently dozens of studies exist that report on the use of iMRI for pituitary tumor resection. Before the use of iMRI, a postoperative MRI within 3 months of surgery was used to determine residual tumor volume. Several studies have compared the iMRI findings to the gold-standard postoperative MRI o define ability of iMRI to detect residual tumor. Of studies where a 0.15-T iMRI was used, sensitivity and specificity was wide ranging, from as low as 32.4% and 62.5% and as high as 97.8% and 100%, respectively.[4–8] This variability is thought to reflect different radiologist and surgeon experience in interpreting iMRI images.

Studies evaluating residual with ≥0.5-T iMRI have been more promising, with consistent sensitivity and sensitivity of 90%.[9–12] Overall, these studies support that magnet strength ≥0.5 T may improve the reliable detection of true tumor residual in intraoperative imaging. However, with improved imaging detail comes an increased need to interpret subtle findings. One study using 1.5-T iMRI suggested that the sensitivity of iMRI for true residual tumor reached 100% if lesions were >3 mm.[13] Fomekong and colleagues[14] looked at 73 cases of pituitary adenomas that were resected using a 3-T iMRI and in 3 cases, the intraoperative imaging results were suspicious for a minor residue but not convincing enough for further surgery. At gold-standard 3-month postoperative MRI, no residual tumor was identified in any of these cases.

Impact of Intraoperative MRI on Extent of Pituitary Tumor Resection

Not surprisingly, with the ability to detect residual tumor with high accuracy, studies of ≥0.5-T iMRI show that the use of the intraoperative imaging

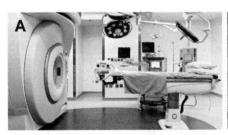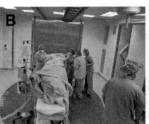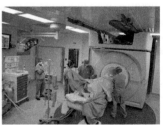

Fig. 1. (A) Massachusetts General Hospital neurosurgical operating room. IMRIS (Deerfield Imaging, Minnetonka, MN) magnet on left moving on ceiling-mounted rails toward the MRI-compatible operating table. (B) Patient is intubated and under general anesthesia on MRI-compatible operating table. Photo on left shows the operating room team preparing the patient before opening the magnet room doors. On right, the team is ensuring safe entry of the patient into the 70-cm bore IMRIS magnet in advance of obtaining intraoperative MR images.

can improve the likelihood of GTR. Actionable residual tumor typically represents tumor that remains within the sellar and suprasellar region that is still accessible with the transsphenoidal technique. Nearly all studies have indicated that, when actionable residual tumor was identified through iMRI, further resection was possible.[15] Further resection occurred in rates from 10% to 83% of cases with iMRI ranging from 0.15 to 1.5 T.[9,14,16] Of note, for all studies iMRI was reported to be performed after the surgeon considered that maximal resection was achieved. However, the vastly varying rates of further resection suggest that, in some cases, it is likely that iMRI was performed as an interval assessment of resection when it was more likely than not that further tumor resection would be necessary.

Studies using 3-T iMRI are more limited because facilities using this magnet strength are a rarity. Nevertheless, in one study by Netuka and colleagues,[17] 85 patients underwent resection with 3-T iMRI whereby it was found that the use of iMRI led to a net 22.4% increase in GTR. In fact, rates of GTR significantly increase in most studies. One large series by Coburger and colleagues[18] compared 67 patients who underwent surgery without iMRI with 76 patients who underwent surgery with 1.5-T iMRI. A GTR was achieved in 73% of non-MRI patients and in 91% of iMRI patients (P<.034).

Of studies that quantified the additional tumor removal, there was an average of 0.9 mL of residual tumor removed.[9,18] Several studies have tracked where residual tumor most commonly occurred in the iMRI. Paternó and Fahlbusch[13] found that, of 72 patients undergoing pituitary adenomas resection with iMRI, tumor remnants most commonly occurred in close proximity to the pituitary stalk (30%), anterior under descending folds of diaphragm sella (30%), and posteriorly (26%).

Intraoperative MRI and Endoscopy for Pituitary Tumors: Comparative and Additive Studies

In addition to the growing use of iMRI, use of endoscopy in transsphenoidal pituitary surgery has also greatly expanded over the last 2 decades.[19] Several studies have compared and contrasted the role of these 2 technologies in identifying tumor and improving resection rates. Most studies indicate that iMRI offers a higher sensitivity and specificity for identifying residual tumor, even in the hands of experienced endoscopic surgeons.[20] One group found that 1.5-T iMRI had a sensitivity and specificity for tumor of 100% compared with 21% and 78% for

endoscopy.[9] A group from the University of Cincinnati were early adopters and proponents of the iMRI, reporting in 2001 on usefulness in improving extent of resection in 30 microscopic transsphenoidal cases.[21] By 2010, their group reported that in a series of 27 patients undergoing resection with endoscopic technique, the iMRI could identify unexpected residual tumor not found with the endoscope in 15% of cases, and concluded that the use of endoscopy was a good substitute for practitioners without access to iMRI.[16] Common locations of residual tumor not seen with the endoscope included the cavernous sinus, suprasellar space, and areas lateral to the sella.[9,13]

When looking at the endoscopic technique in comparison with microscopic technique, no studies have looked at head-to-head comparison with the iMRI.[22] In a *Neurosurgery Clinics* review, Chittiboina[23] found the iMRI studies in aggregation to have reported a smaller proportion of unexpected residuals with endoscopic technique (34% ± 26%) than those using microscopy (44% ± 18%) for transsphenoidal surgery (P = .04). In a large retrospective series of 446 transsphenoidal pituitary cases, Sylvester and colleagues[24] demonstrated that the endoscopic technique with iMRI was associated with higher extent of resection than with the microscopic technique (odds ratio 2.05, 95% confidence interval 1.21–3.46, P<.01), and was associated with a higher odds of increased extent of resection status than either endoscopy without iMRI or microscopy with iMRI.

Intraoperative MRI for Functioning Adenomas

Although most studies have focused their analysis on the role of iMRI for nonfunctioning adenomas, there have been a few reports of outcomes for functional tumors and the effect of iMRI on remission rates. Fahlbusch and colleagues[25] prospectively studied 23 patients with acromegaly who underwent first-time transsphenoidal surgery using a 1.5-T iMRI. They reported that, for cases in which complete resection was thought possible, iMRI helped improve remission rates from 33% to 44%. Another group looked at the usefulness of 1.5-T iMRI for a series of 14 patients with functioning microadenomas with maximum tumor diameter of 9.3 ± 2.6 mm.[26] They found that the overall long-term endocrine remission rate was 78.5% instead of the 57.1% it might have been without the additional resection performed following iMRI.

Among 66 cases of functional tumor resection using iMRI, Sylvester and colleagues[24] found that there was significantly lower extent of resection in functioning tumors compared with nonfunctioning tumors. Whether this reflects the more aggressive, and therefore invasive, nature of functioning tumors was not specifically analyzed, but this remains the hypothesis. There was no change in biochemical remission rates between cases done with or without iMRI. The authors' center continues to use iMRI for most functioning tumors except for MRI-negative corticotropin-secreting tumors.

COMPLICATIONS AND OUTCOMES

As with the introduction of any new surgical technology, the use if iMRI and its effect on patient safety is important and has been well studied. No studies have noted significant adverse events related to iMRI or accidents caused by the ferromagnetic instruments. At the authors' center, in more than 500 transsphenoidal cases using iMRI no adverse events have been recorded and the surgical workflow is typically interrupted for 30 minutes to obtain images. Other than technical complications that might be posed by iMRI, one might also wonder whether finding residual tumor on intraoperative imaging might result in overzealous exploration leading to worsened postoperative morbidity. Studies have fortunately indicated that this is not the case.[12,15,26,27]

Visual Outcomes

Compression of the optic nerves and/or chiasm is a common surgical indication for patients undergoing transsphenoidal surgery, and, as a result, the role of iMRI has been well studied for its role in aiding visual recovery. In one series, Berkmann and colleagues[28] studied 32 patients who presented with visual deficits and found that 1.5-T iMRI finding of optic apparatus decompression was predictive of recovery in 100% of patients within 1 month postoperatively. In a review of several studies that examined visual outcomes after transsphenoidal surgery, including 5 studies in which iMRI had been used, the investigators found that iMRI safely increased the resection of pituitary macroadenomas remnants that were poorly visualized by microscopic technique.[11,25,29–32]

Endocrine Outcomes

Given the nature of pituitary tumor surgery involving surgical dissection within or adjacent to normal glands, one concern is whether use of iMRI influences postoperative hormonal outcomes. Many studies have retrospectively analyzed hormonal outcomes and have largely found no significant risk to postoperative endocrine function or recovery. In an analysis of 92 patients, Berkmann and colleagues[4] found the incidence of new-onset pituitary deficits to be 29% in the iMRI group and 45% in the control group, with no significant difference in rates of diabetes insipidus. In a study of 133 patients iMRI allowed for a significantly increased rate of GTR, but this was not associated with an increased incidence of postoperative hypopituitarism or lower recovery rates in the pituitary axes (both $P>.05$).[33]

Long-Term Outcomes

Because of the relatively recent introduction and adaptation of iMRI in the late 1990s and early 2000s and the slow-growing nature of these tumors, there remain limited data on the impact of long-term control rates with and without iMRI. In a retrospective review of 143 patients, Coburger and colleagues[18] found that GTR was achieved in 91% of iMRI patients and 73% of non-iMRI patients, and that at 2-year follow-up this translated to a higher progression-free survival in the iMRI group. Other groups have also found that with longer-term follow-up, the iMRI group had lower rates of recurrence and, furthermore, there was need for further therapy (radiosurgery or resection) in no-one with iMRI versus 13% of the non-iMRI patients ($P = .013$).[4,9] As the use of iMRI continues, future studies will be able to study longer-term follow-up of progression-free survival, reoperation rates, need for further therapy, and remission from hormone-secreting tumors.

CASE EXAMPLES

This section describes 3 patients from the Massachusetts General Hospital Pituitary and Neuroendocrine Clinical Center who underwent transsphenoidal surgery using 3-T iMRI on the IMRIS system.

Case 1

A 63-year-old woman presented with several months of vision change, and was found to have dense bitemporal hemianopia on neuro-ophthalmology examination. MRI of pituitary demonstrated a large sellar and suprasellar lesion with optic chiasm compression (**Fig. 2**A). There was some suggestion of cavernous sinus invasion, so the ability to achieve GTR was unknown. Endocrine evaluation revealed it as a nonfunctioning tumor. Transsphenoidal surgery using microscopic technique and endoscopic assist was used for the surgery, and iMRI revealed no obvious residual and a decompressed optic chiasm (**Fig. 2**B). The surgery was completed following completion and

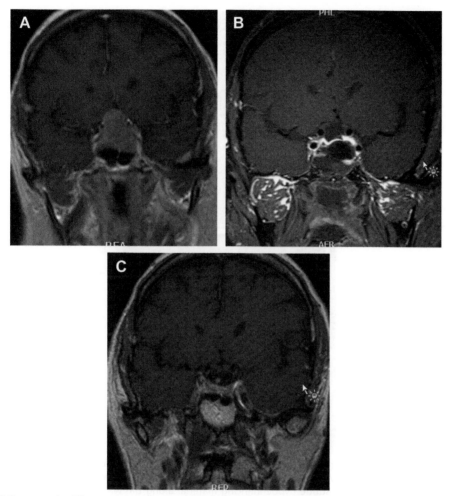

Fig. 2. (*A*) Preoperative T1-postcontrast coronal MR image demonstrating a large sellar lesion with suprasellar extension and compression of the optic chiasm. (*B*) Intraoperative T1-postcontrast coronal MRI demonstrating normal enhancing gland to the left of the sella and fat packing within the sella, with no obvious residual tumor. The optic chiasm is decompressed. (*C*) Postoperative T1-postcontrast coronal MR image demonstrating no residual tumor within the sella or suprasellar region and a decompressed optic chiasm.

radiologic interpretation of the imaging. A 6-week postoperative MRI confirmed a GTR of the tumor (**Fig. 2**C). At this visit the patient's vision had returned to normal based on repeat neuro-ophthalmologic evaluation.

Case 2

A 59-year-old woman presented with nearly 1 year of intermittent headache, dizziness, changes in her voice, and difficulty swallowing over the last 8 to 9 months. MRI of pituitary demonstrated a macro-adenoma within the right side of the gland with no obvious invasion of the cavernous sinus or supra-sellar region (**Fig. 3**A). Endocrine evaluation revealed an insulin-like growth factor-1 (IGF-1) level of 708 ng/mL (normal 44–240 ng/mL). Trans-sphenoidal surgery using microscopic technique was used for the surgery and iMRI was obtained

(**Fig. 3**B). The radiologist considered that there was a hypoenhancing portion adjacent to the right wall of the cavernous sinus, suspicious for resid-ual. Therefore, the resection cavity was re-explored and further curettage yielded no further material consistent with tumor. A 6-week postop-erative MRI confirmed GTR of the tumor (**Fig. 3**C). At 3-month endocrine follow-up, her IGF-1 had normalized to 177 ng/mL.

Case 3

A 36-year-old woman presented with 6 months of vision change, and was found to have dense bitemporal hemianopia with mild dyschromatop-sia. MRI of pituitary demonstrated a large sellar and suprasellar lesion with optic chiasm compres-sion and bilateral cavernous sinus invasion (**Fig. 4**A). Endocrine evaluation revealed it as a

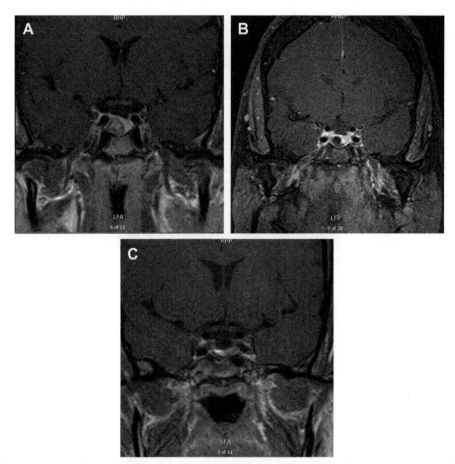

Fig. 3. (*A*) Preoperative T1-postcontrast coronal MR image demonstrating a right-sided sellar lesion. (*B*) Intraoperative T1-postcontrast coronal MR image demonstrating normal enhancing gland to the left of the sella and fat packing within the sella, with subtle hypoenhancing material along the wall of the right cavernous sinus. (*C*) Postoperative T1-postcontrast coronal MR image demonstrating no residual tumor within the sella or suprasellar region, and a resorbing fat graft.

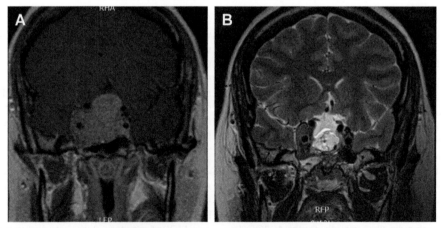

Fig. 4. (*A*) Preoperative T1-postcontrast coronal MR image demonstrating a large sellar lesion with suprasellar extension, invasion into right and left cavernous sinus, and compression of the optic chiasm. (*B*) Intraoperative T1-postcontrast coronal MR image demonstrating residual tumor in the right cavernous sinus, fat packing within the sella, with no obvious actionable residual tumor in the sella. The optic chiasm is decompressed.

nonfunctioning tumor. Transsphenoidal surgery using microscopic technique was used for the surgery and iMRI was obtained. Images revealed that the tumor within the sella and suprasellar space had been resected, and the remaining tumor appeared to be greater in the right than left cavernous sinuses (**Fig. 4**B). Given decompression of the optic chiasm and no actionable remaining tumor within the sella, the surgery was completed following completion and radiologic interpretation of the imaging. A 6-week postoperative MRI showed stable tumor in the cavernous sinus, with no tumor within the sella.

SUMMARY

Overall, the use of iMRI in transsphenoidal surgery for pituitary adenomas has been proved to be safe and effective and shows promise for more long-standing effects on improved tumor-growth control rates and remission from functioning tumors. At the authors' center, as illustrated by the case examples, 3-T iMRI is used for a variety of reasons. Most commonly, the iMRI allows assessment of residual tumor, as well as decompression of the optic apparatus in cases of large tumors or compressive cystic lesions. iMRI is also used for assistance with intraoperative guidance in cases with challenging anatomy, albeit with much less frequency than for the other indications.

The literature supports that the use of iMRI increases the rates of GTR using both endoscopic and microscopic techniques, and studies with the longest follow-up show that this translates into higher rates of progression-free survival and lower rates of radiation therapy. The Congress of Neurologic Surgeons 2016 guidelines agreed that iMRI, whether low-field or high-field, helps improve immediate overall GTR of nonfunctioning pituitary adenomas.[34] It will be interesting to study long-term follow-up in the decades ahead as more cases are analyzed and the experience with iMRI grows among surgeons and radiologists. Although there is additional upfront cost in performing iMRI, this may translate into reduced overall costs over the long term if its use decreases repeat surgery, radiation therapy, or medication therapy. Studies of such cost-effectiveness and tumor control rates will no doubt serve the field tremendously in the years ahead.

REFERENCES

1. Liu JK, Cohen-Gadol AA, Laws ER, et al. Harvey Cushing and Oskar Hirsch: early forefathers of modern transsphenoidal surgery. J Neurosurg 2005;103:1096–104.

2. Brochier S, Galland F, Kujas M, et al. Factors predicting relapse of nonfunctioning pituitary macroadenomas after neurosurgery: a study of 142 patients. Eur J Endocrinol 2010;163:193–200.

3. Mislow JMK, Golby AJ, Black PM. Origins of intraoperative MRI. Magn Reson Imaging Clin N Am 2010;18:1–10.

4. Berkmann S, Fandino J, Müller B, et al. Intraoperative MRI and endocrinological outcome of transsphenoidal surgery for non-functioning pituitary adenoma. Acta Neurochir 2012;154:639–47.

5. Kim EH, Oh MC, Kim SH. Application of low-field intraoperative magnetic resonance imaging in transsphenoidal surgery for pituitary adenomas: technical points to improve the visibility of the tumor resection margin. Acta Neurochir 2013;155:485–93.

6. Hlavica M, Bellut D, Lemm D, et al. Impact of ultra-low-field intraoperative magnetic resonance imaging on extent of resection and frequency of tumor recurrence in 104 surgically treated nonfunctioning pituitary adenomas. World Neurosurg 2013;79:99–109.

7. Wu J-S, Shou X-F, Yao C-J, et al. Transsphenoidal pituitary macroadenomas resection guided by polestar N20 low-field intraoperative magnetic resonance imaging. Neurosurgery 2009;65:63–71.

8. Narang KS, Jha AN. Intraoperative imaging in neurosurgery. London: JP Medical Ltd; 2017.

9. Berkmann S, Schlaffer S, Nimsky C, et al. Follow-up and long-term outcome of nonfunctioning pituitary adenoma operated by transsphenoidal surgery with intraoperative high-field magnetic resonance imaging. Acta Neurochir 2014;156:2233–43 [discussion: 2243].

10. Vitaz TW, Inkabi KE, Carrubba CJ. Intraoperative MRI for transphenoidal procedures: short-term outcome for 100 consecutive cases. Clin Neurol Neurosurg 2011;113:731–5.

11. Nimsky C, Keller BV, Ganslandt O, et al. Intraoperative high-field magnetic resonance imaging in transsphenoidal surgery of hormonally inactive pituitary macroadenomas. Neurosurgery 2006;59:105–14.

12. Ramm-Pettersen J, Berg-Johnsen J, Hol PK, et al. Intra-operative MRI facilitates tumour resection during trans-sphenoidal surgery for pituitary adenomas. Acta Neurochir 2011;153:1367–73.

13. Paternó V, Fahlbusch R. High-Field iMRI in transsphenoidal pituitary adenoma surgery with special respect to typical localization of residual tumor. Acta Neurochir (Wein) 2014;156:463–74.

14. Fomekong E, Duprez T, Docquier M-A, et al. Intraoperative 3T MRI for pituitary macroadenoma resection: Initial experience in 73 consecutive patients. Clin Neurol Neurosurg 2014;126:143–9.

15. Patel KS, Yao Y, Wang R, et al. Intraoperative magnetic resonance imaging assessment of nonfunctioning pituitary adenomas during transsphenoidal surgery. Pituitary 2016;19:222–31.

16. Theodosopoulos PV, Leach J, Kerr RG, et al. Maximizing the extent of tumor resection during transsphenoidal surgery for pituitary macroadenomas: can endoscopy replace intraoperative magnetic resonance imaging? J Neurosurg 2010;112:736–43.

17. Netuka D, Masopust V, Belšán T, et al. One year experience with 3.0 T intraoperative MRI in pituitary surgery. Acta Neurochir Suppl 2011;109:157–9.

18. Coburger J, König R, Seitz K, et al. Determining the utility of intraoperative magnetic resonance imaging for transsphenoidal surgery: a retrospective study. J Neurosurg 2014;120:346–56.

19. Rolston JD, Han SJ, Aghi MK. Nationwide shift from microscopic to endoscopic transsphenoidal pituitary surgery. Pituitary 2016;19:248–50.

20. Zaidi HA, De Los Reyes K, Barkhoudarian G, et al. The utility of high-resolution intraoperative MRI in endoscopic transsphenoidal surgery for pituitary macroadenomas: early experience in the advanced multimodality image guided operating suite. Neurosurg Focus 2016;40:E18.

21. Bohinski RJ, Warnick RE, Gaskill-Shipley MF, et al. Intraoperative magnetic resonance imaging to determine the extent of resection of pituitary macroadenomas during transsphenoidal microsurgery. Neurosurgery 2001;49:1133–43 [discussion: 1143–4].

22. Almutairi RD, Muskens IS, Cote DJ, et al. Gross total resection of pituitary adenomas after endoscopic vs. microscopic transsphenoidal surgery: a meta-analysis. Acta Neurochir 2018;160:1005–21.

23. Chittiboina P. iMRI during transsphenoidal surgery. Neurosurg Clin N Am 2017;28:499–512.

24. Sylvester PT, Evans JA, Zipfel GJ, et al. Combined high-field intraoperative magnetic resonance imaging and endoscopy increase extent of resection and progression-free survival for pituitary adenomas. Pituitary 2015;18:72–85.

25. Fahlbusch R, Keller B v, Ganslandt O, et al. Transsphenoidal surgery in acromegaly investigated by intraoperative high-field magnetic resonance imaging. Eur J Endocrinol 2005;153:239–48.

26. Tanei T, Nagatani T, Nakahara N, et al. Use of high-field intraoperative magnetic resonance imaging during endoscopic transsphenoidal surgery for functioning pituitary microadenomas and small adenomas located in the intrasellar region. Neurol Med Chir 2013;53:501–10.

27. Anand VK, Schwartz TH, Hiltzik DH, et al. Endoscopic transsphenoidal pituitary surgery with real-time intraoperative magnetic resonance imaging. Am J Rhinol 2006;20:401–5.

28. Berkmann S, Fandino J, Zosso S, et al. Intraoperative magnetic resonance imaging and early prognosis for vision after transsphenoidal surgery for sellar lesions. J Neurosurg 2011;115:518–27.

29. Jones J, Ruge J. Intraoperative magnetic resonance imaging in pituitary macroadenoma surgery: an assessment of visual outcome. Neurosurg Focus 2007;23:E12.

30. Fahlbusch R, Ganslandt O, Buchfelder M, et al. Intraoperative magnetic resonance imaging during transsphenoidal surgery. J Neurosurg 2001;95:381–90.

31. Pergolizzi RS Jr, Schwartz RB, Hsu L, et al. Transsphenoidal pituitary resection with intraoperative MR guidance: preliminary results. In: Ryan TP, Wong TZ, editors. SPIE Proceedings volume 3594. Thermal treatment of tissue with image guidance. 1999. https://doi.org/10.1117/12.348742.

32. Nimsky C, Ganslandt O, Von Keller B, et al. Intraoperative high-field-strength MR imaging: implementation and experience in 200 patients. Radiology 2004;233:67–78.

33. Zhibin Z, Peng W, Shiyu F, et al. Endocrinological outcomes of intraoperative MRI-guided endoscopic transsphenoidal surgery for non-functioning pituitary adenoma. Turk Neurosurg 2018. https://doi.org/10.5137/1019-5149.JTN.22603-18.2.

34. Kuo JS, Barkhoudarian G, Farrell CJ, et al. Congress of neurological surgeons systematic review and evidence-based guideline on surgical techniques and technologies for the management of patients with nonfunctioning pituitary adenomas. Neurosurgery 2016;79:E536–8.

The Role of Three-Dimensional Endoscopy in Pituitary Adenoma Surgery

Kumar Vasudevan, MD*, Hassan Saad, MD, Nelson M. Oyesiku, MD, PhD

KEYWORDS

- 3D endoscopy • Endoscopic endonasal surgery • Pituitary adenoma surgery

KEY POINTS

- The recent introduction of 3D endoscopes in pituitary adenoma surgery aims to improve visualization and understanding of anatomy during these complex procedures.
- 3D endoscopes have theoretic advantages over 2D in stereoscopic vision, visualizing tumor around neurovascular structures, and repairing postoperative cerebrospinal fluid leaks.
- Disadvantages of 3D endoscopes include higher system cost, larger scope size, need for accessory equipment, and strict requirements for operating position must be considered.
- Multiple preclinical, clinical, and cadaveric studies have shown 3D endoscopy to have noninferior outcomes to 2D work in terms of complication rates, learning curve, and outcomes.
- Our and other groups' experiences with 3D endoscopy suggest that, with growing use, it will soon become the standard of care of endoscopic pituitary surgery.

The advent of transsphenoidal approach to the sella represented a major step forward in the treatment of pituitary adenomas and other sellar and parasellar pathology. In his seminal paper describing the successful surgical treatment of an acromegaly patient via a transfacial, transsphenoidal approach, Cushing[1] remarked that it "was surprising to find how small an opening had actually been made through the ethmoidal region and how accessible the sella turcica actually proved to be after the landmarks had once been well determined." The continued evolution of this technique led several years later to the near-contemporaneous development of the sublabial and transnasal microscopic approaches by Cushing and Oskar Hirsch.[2] Key to the success of the transsphenoidal approach was its minimal invasiveness, but many surgeons found the lack of illumination and visualization of parasellar neurovascular structures to be limiting.

The development of the endoscopic endonasal transsphenoidal approach to the sella (EES) revitalized the use of this corridor to treat a wide variety of lesions. Modern endoscopes provide unparalleled views past the nasal passages into the sphenoid sinus, and the wide variety of endoscopic instruments have offered improvements in soft tissue exposure, bone removal, tumor dissection, and hemostasis, which make microsurgery feasible. Classically, EES has used 2-dimensional (2D) endoscopes. The recent development of 3-dimensional (3D) endoscopy (3DE) improves on the depth of vision offered by 2D systems, and may improve visualization of the critical structures involved in EES. As 3D scopes have become increasingly compact and higher-resolution, many centers have advocated for its use to improve resection rates; decrease complications, such as vascular injury and cerebrospinal fluid (CSF) leak; and lessen the learning curve for

Disclosure Statement: The authors have nothing to disclose.
Department of Neurosurgery, Emory University, 1365-B Clifton Road, 6th Floor, Atlanta, GA 30322, USA
* Corresponding author.
E-mail address: KVasud2@emory.edu

Neurosurg Clin N Am 30 (2019) 421–432
https://doi.org/10.1016/j.nec.2019.05.012
1042-3680/19/

performing EES and pituitary adenoma surgery.[3] Because of the real costs associated with dedicated 3DE equipment, and some possible disadvantages of this approach, an honest appraisal of the value of 3D for EES is essential. Here we discuss the development of 3D endoscopes, address the advantages and disadvantages of using them, review recent studies of EES outcomes using 3D endoscopes, and discuss our personal experience with 3DE.

DEVELOPMENT OF NEUROENDOSCOPY AND THE TRANSSPHENOIDAL APPROACH

Speculums and tubular instruments for intranasal examination reached a point of maturity in 1859, when Czermak mounted a mirror to the end of a small-diameter rod to visualize the posterior nasopharynx and oropharynx,[4] and the field of "rhinoscopy" was born. Several small modifications over the next few decades continued to improve visualization and soft tissue retraction. The popularization of cocaine as a vasoconstrictor, in particular, enabled more intranasal access without excessive blood loss. Coupled with a head mirror for reflecting environmental light into the deep nasal cavity, nineteenth century endoscopists could perform basic anterior and posterior rhinoscopic procedures. But proper illumination and visualization still remained a challenge.[5] Urologists, who were concurrently devising methods to examine the urethra and bladder, were the first to move the modes of magnification and illumination closer to the field, a step that proved critical. Building on the work of Bozzini and his "Lichtleiter" in the early 1800s, in 1853 Antonin Desormeaux of France first coined the term "endoscope" for his device, which used lenses to focus light from a continuously burning lamp at the opposite end of the instrument.[4] German urologist Maximillian Nitze revolutionized the device by realizing that, "to light up a room one must carry the lamp inside"[6]: he placed the lens and light source close to the tip of a long instrument and visualization improved. This was made safer when Nitze used Thomas Edison's incandescent light to create a filamentous light source that could be threaded through the scope itself.

By the 1920s, the endoscope had begun to be used by Dandy and other neurosurgeons for intraventricular procedures, whereas the transsphenoidal route to the sella was being explored by Cushing and Hirsch on both sides of the Atlantic.[4] By the end of his career, however, Cushing had all but abandoned it in favor of the transcranial route, which he believed offered superior visualization, vascular control, and visual outcomes, and the

transsphenoidal approach fell out of favor for the next several decades.[7] The 1960s allowed key advances that revived interest in EES, among them the use of image intensification and radiofluoroscopy. Jules Hardy's use of the surgical microscope beginning in 1967 allowed him to accumulate a large series of fluoroscopic-guided transsphenoidal microscopic hypophysectomies, and to reinvigorate interest in the transsphenoidal route.[8] By the 1990s, neurosurgeons observed the expanded field of view and up-close anatomic views afforded to endoscopic sinus surgeons and began to use endoscopes as an adjunct to microscopic transsphenoidal pituitary adenoma surgery. In 1996, Carrau and Jho, an otolaryngologist and neurosurgeon, first reported the purely endoscopic approach[9] that has become the standard for EES.

THE SWITCH TO ENDOSCOPIC ENDONASAL TRANSSPHENOIDAL APPROACH TO THE SELLA

Endoscopic approaches are well-suited to pituitary adenoma surgery; they solve several issues that hampered early surgeons' efforts to approach the sella without violating the calvarium. Approaching the sphenoid sinus necessitates manipulation of the soft tissues of the nose. The instruments of early rhinologists were used to somewhat blindly perform these maneuvers, often leading to suboptimal visualization. The vascularity of these structures and inability to visualize sources of bleeding often made hemostasis a limiting factor. The variability of nasal soft tissue anatomy often necessitates accessory procedures during EES, such as septoplasty or resection/reduction of hypertrophied turbinates. Most centers now perform preoperative endoscopic endonasal screening to anticipate and prepare for these issues.[10]

The sellar region is a remarkably dense tangle of neurovascular structures separated by folds of dura and ridges of bone.[11] Transcranial routes held favor here because they allowed visualization of these structures, vascular control in the event of injury, freedom of dissection to mobilize delicate nerves, and room for using multiple instruments within the field. They allowed for the easy use of the operating microscope and its stereoscopic vision. Early surgeons had to trade limited visualization of intrasellar contents for better visualization of structures at risk. Infrasellar approaches to pituitary adenomas were appealing because they allowed for more direct access to the pathology and visualization of blood supply to vital structures, such as the optic chiasm. They were overall less morbid, and were ideal for intrasellar pituitary macroadenomas or functional microadenomas that otherwise were poorly visualized from a suprasellar approach, but technical limitations made infrasellar access difficult.

A confluence of new developments on several fronts led to the adoption of EES as the preferred approach to pituitary adenomas. The development of the videoendoscope, particularly bringing the imaging element closer to the pathology, was crucial in widening the field of view to the lateral structures and increased safety. New endoscopic instruments made it possible to perform true microneurosurgery through the nose. An enhanced understanding of pituitary anatomy and adenoma pathology, particularly patterns of cavernous sinus invasion and the development of the pseudocapsular technique of resection, suited for the scope.[12] Neurosurgeons have become more familiar with endoscopic approaches and sellar anatomy from below. Learning and knowledge creation in endoscopic pituitary surgery has become organized. Neurosurgeons who were used to the operating microscope are learning to adapt their techniques to 2D endoscopic views. 3D endoscopes may represent the next step, allowing for the stereoscopic benefits of microscopic surgery with the distinct advantages of endoscopy discussed here.

MODERN THREE-DIMENSIONAL ENDOSCOPY

The introduction of 3DE represents the next logical step in the evolution of EES. Modern endoscopes perform two key functions. The first is illumination, which in modern systems is conveyed from a central light source through optical fibers in the outermost layer of the endoscope rod assembly. The second is image capture, originally performed by a rod-lens system, now performed by a camera mounted to the end of the scope. In traditional 2D endoscopy, a single ocular provides 2D image capture that is projected on a single monitor for use by the operating surgeon.[13] One struggle of the last several decades of endoscope development has been containing both of these functions, in addition to working and irrigating channels, into a device of sufficiently small caliber. Most modern 2D endoscopes range in diameter from 2 mm to 6 mm, requiring absolute precision engineering to meet needed specifications.

Rather than truly projecting in three dimensions, 3D images are typically created by forcing the perception of depth in 2D images. Stereoscopy is the most common way to do this, and involves presenting slightly different (usually horizontally displaced) images to each eye such that higher visual processing interpolates them as an image with depth. Stereoscopic effects are triggered in modern cinemas and televisions by separating the images by color layers, polarization, or even active shuttering of one eye at a time.[14] "Stereoendoscopes" long sought to replicate these properties with two separate rod-lens or camera assemblies capturing different images, but these require large scopes and produces substandard 3D images, and until recently were all but abandoned in neuroendoscopy.[3]

The latest 3D endoscopes aim to refine the principles of stereoendoscopy with modern engineering and intelligent visual processing. Some models replicate the dual-camera, dual-chip assembly (eg, ENDOEYE FLEX 3D, Olympus, Tokyo, Japan) with accompanying polarized eyeglasses. Only with recently developed image sensors have endoscope diameters of less than 1 cm been achievable in these models. A recent, widely adopted model (Visionsense Ltd, Petach Tikva, Israel) uses a single chip with a large array of microlenses in an "insect eye" array. A single object is viewed through dual pupils and a single lens, then redirected by the microlens array to generate two slightly different images **(Fig. 1)**. This produces a more accurate

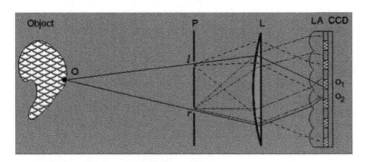

Fig. 1. Diagram representation of the "insect eye" system for generating 3D endoscopic images. The single lens (L) receives image data via two pupil openings (l and r) in a single focal plane (P). The charge-coupled device (CCD) contains an array of microlenses (LA). Rays focused through each of the pupil openings (*dashed* and *dotted lines*) are emitted toward the lens array and focused by the array onto pixels at the contralateral aspect of the CCD. This generates two slightly different images, creating a stereoscopic depth effect after post-processing by the system. (*From* Tabaee A, Anand VK, Fraser JF, et al. Three-dimensional endoscopic pituitary surgery. Neurosurgery 2009;64(5 Suppl 2):288-293; with permission.)

stereoscopic effect because of the single ocular, and enables a scope diameter of 4 mm.[15] The newer Multiangle, Rear-Viewing Endoscopic Tool (MARVEL, California Institute of Technology, Pasadena, California, USA) also uses a single lens and small diameter. Stereopsis is created by a "complementary multibandpass filter" in each eye that filters light of a certain wavelength; this setup allows for a single pupil, single lens, and customizable angle of the scope (**Fig. 2**).[16]

ADVANTAGES AND DISADVANTAGES OF THREE-DIMENSIONAL ENDOSCOPY

The impairment of depth perception from 2D endoscopes can possibly lead to poor eye-hand coordination, image distortion, difficulty in executing precise movements, reduced ability to estimate size, and deterioration of accuracy and efficiency.[17–20] The 2D system has also been criticized for reduced sharpness and clarity, and a steeper learning curve.[3,19,21] An essential part of training is developing skills that compensate for this lack of stereoscopy, including visual and tactile cues to simulate depth and learning the appearance of key structures from a coronal, 2D vantage point. The skill set required is fairly divorced from those taught to most neurosurgeons and requires a large number of cases to master. The Pittsburgh group has proposed a stepwise progression of skills and case difficulty in endoscopic endonasal surgery,[22] and learning these compensatory skills is critical to progression.

For numerous reasons, 3D endoscopes may offer a more shallow learning curve than 2D ones.[23–25] 3D has the advantage of improved depth perception.[26] This can aid in recognizing layers of dissection and understanding neurovascular relationships,[27] particularly when dealing with tumors with suprasellar extension.[28] These visualization advantages could help to decrease CSF leak rates, although this has not been shown to be the case in several case series comparing pituitary surgery outcomes using 2D versus 3D endoscopes (discussed later).[3,19] In their series of 70 patients that included 42 pituitary adenomas, Catapano and colleagues[29] reported that the use of 3D high-definition (HD) endoscope rendered their surgeries safer and allowed the use of "microsurgery technique" that was similar to that provided by a microscope, such as working behind and around neurovascular structures and identifying tissue planes for dissection in 3D space.

But the adoption of modern 3D endoscopes has been slow and limited. Many of their limitations are particular to the mode of 3D projection; most published experience is with the stereoscopic, two-display version. Commonly cited is a smaller field of view, which is reduced by as much as 52%, possibly secondary to a small "virtual interpupillary distance" between the two oculars.[30] Other pitfalls are issues with sharpness, brightness, and contrast of the image, in addition to ghosting, ocular fatigue and strain, headaches, nausea and dizziness.[15,31–33] Data on newer, single chip models are lacking. The lack of angled 3D scopes is another barrier, because surgeons have to switch to angled 2D endoscopes when required.[32] The stereoscopic 3D lens has also been noted to be more sensitive to soiling.[3,32,34] Some 3D screens displayed excessive red color saturation, which is problematic when multiple bleeding points are present in a narrow surgical corridor.[15] Some of these early limitations were addressed and overcome in new generations of 3D endoscopes.[30,35]

A   **B**

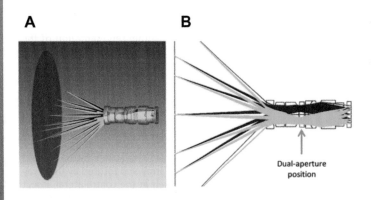

Dual-aperture position

Fig. 2. Imaging basis for the novel Multiangle, Rear-Viewing Endoscopic Tool (MARVEL). The stereo camera is housed (*A*) in a single lens, dual aperture system that minimizes space requirements. The viewpoints are distinguished using complementary multibandpass filters, which are coated over each aperture and create transmission bands (*B*) whose wavelengths are complementary. This creates two slightly different images, which imparts stereoscopic properties to the image, simulating depth perception. (*From* Bae SY, Korniski RJ, Shearn M, et al. 4-mm-diameter three-dimensional imaging endoscope with steerable camera for minimally invasive surgery (3-D-MARVEL). Neurophotonics 2017;4(1):011008; with permission.)

Additional limitations include that some 3D endoscopes are wide in diameter, which decreases maneuverability in narrow spaces.[34,36] The screen must be positioned exactly orthogonally from the operator to best appreciate the 3D images, which is an issue in small surgical suites.[19] Ophthalmologic conditions, such as strabismus, amblyopia, and optic nerve hypoplasia, can make certain individuals incapable of appreciating 3D images. The need for special glasses, along with the higher cost of 3D endoscopic systems, must be acknowledged.[29,36] The higher price is attributed not only to the 3D endoscope itself, but also to the fact that most 2D systems share hardware resources with several other endoscopic systems used by other specialties, such as urology or general surgery.[15] Although these costs are likely to decrease over time, institutions performing fewer EES cases may not be able to justify them in the short term.

THREE-DIMENSIONAL ENDOSCOPES FOR ENDOSCOPIC ENDONASAL TRANSSPHENOIDAL APPROACH TO THE SELLA: PRECLINICAL STUDIES

Several cadaveric and simulated-environment studies have been conducted to evaluate the use of 3D endoscopes for EES for adenomas. **Table 1** summarizes the cadaveric studies. Roth and colleagues[7] and Beer-Furlan and coworkers[37] used the 2D and 3D endoscopic systems to illustrate their visualization of complex neurovascular structures and to present their experience with the new 3D system. They found that 3DE enhanced depth perception and appreciation of anatomic relationships, which increased manual dexterity and allowed for easier dissections. In a subsequent study comparing 2D and 3D, Ogino-Nishimura and coworkers[27] validated these findings and showed, via a questionnaire, that most EES surgeons agreed that 3D endoscopes provided better understanding of surgical anatomy and decreased the rate of complications; most said they would prefer to use 3D endoscopes in clinical settings. They concluded that 3DE was superior to 2D because it enhanced precision and facilitated understanding of posterior nasal structures.

2D and 3D modalities have been compared in preclinical settings under more controlled conditions, mostly with surgeon participants ranging from novices,[38,39] to experts,[40] or a combination of the two.[35,41,42] Anatomic models used ranged from simpler computational ones[30,42,43] to more complex, anatomically correct EES approaches.[40,44] The results of these studies are illustrated in **Table 2**. The outcome measures most frequently analyzed were the execution time of different tasks and number of errors.[41,42] Inoue and colleagues[44] introduced an optical tracking system to analyze the trajectories of endoscopes and study operators' movements.[41] Across all studies, execution time to complete different tasks was either similar between the 2D and 3D groups[35,40,42,43] or decreased in the 3D group.[38,39,41,44] Similarly, 3DE lowered the margin of error in some studies,[35,38,39,41] while not

| Table 1 | | | | |
| Cadaveric studies | | | | |
Author, Year	N	Comparison	Outcome Measures	Outcome
Roth et al,[7] 2009	10 specimens	3D	Qualitative description of benefits of 3D endoscopy	Enhanced depth of perception and spatial orientation
Beer-Furlan et al,[37] 2014	10 specimens	3D	Description of added benefits of 3D endoscopes over 2D endoscopic systems	Enhanced depth perception, high resolution, better identification of anatomic structures, facilitates dissection
Ogino-Nishimura et al,[27] 2015	5 surgeon participants	3D vs 2D	Questionnaire	3D superior for understanding anatomy and decreasing complications Most clinicians want to use 3D in clinical setting: 50% said it makes surgical procedures easier, most said that skull base surgery is where 3D would be most useful

Table 2
Simulated environment studies

Author, Year	Number of Participants	Simulation	Comparison	Outcome Measures	Outcomes
Shah et al,[42] 2011	15	Task design (nerve hook)	3D vs 2D	Execution time, number of errors in different tasks	No difference except for novice users
Inoue et al,[44] 2013	43	Task design (3D skull)	2DHD vs 3DHD	Total path length, execution time, subjective depth perception, and side effects from using the 3D system	3D endoscope superior in tasks requiring depth perception
Kawanishi et al,[39] 2013	30	Task design	2DHD vs 3DHD	Speed, accuracy	Less inaccuracy and execution time with 3D endoscopes All participants preferred 3D endoscopes and none complained of headaches, eyes strain, or other discomfort
Marcus et al,[38] 2014	10	Task design	2D vs 3D and SD vs HD	Speed, accuracy, questionnaire about image quality and perception	Time to task completion was significantly less when using 3D, accuracy greater when using HD; 3D enhanced depth perception, HD enhanced image quality, both improved the likelihood of using the modality again
Van Gompel et al,[30] 2014	1	Simulation chamber	2DHD vs 3D	Field of view	52% reduction of field of view when using 3D endoscope
Raheja et al,[43] 2016	8	Task design	2DHD vs 3DHD	Accuracy, efficiency, speed	In simple tasks, reduced inaccuracy with 3D No difference in complex motor tasks
Rampinelli et al,[41] 2017	68	Task design	2DHD vs 3D	Execution time, jitter analysis, questionnaire	Novices experienced some dizziness and discomfort with 3D, but preferred them overall Shorter execution time and lower error rate with 3D Possible advantage for 3D in jitter (not significant)

(continued on next page)

Table 2
(continued)

Author, Year	Number of Participants	Simulation	Comparison	Outcome Measures	Outcomes
Nassimizadeh et al,[34] 2015	35	Modified box-trainer task (peg transfer)	2DHD vs 3DHD	Time to complete task, adjustment time, past pointing, number of drops, subjective depth perception, field of view, image quality, maneuverability	No difference in time to complete task and adjustment time, depth perception Image quality improved along with reduced past pointing in 3DHD, 77% of operators preferred 3DHD, field of vision reduced in 3DHD

affecting it in others.[40,43] A faster learning curve for trainees using 3DE was demonstrated in several studies,[38,39,43,44] but not in others.[41] Subjective complaints of dizziness and discomfort were reported in small percentages in the nonexpert group in two studies. Marcus and colleagues[38] aimed to study 3D versus 2D and HD versus standard definition simultaneously. They found that the 3DE decreased the task execution time and subjectively enhanced depth perception, whereas HD improved task accuracy and subjectively augmented image quality. They concluded that 3D and HD neuroendoscopy enhance surgical performance in distinct, yet, complimentary ways. 3D endoscopes were the preferred modality in most participants in most preclinical studies.[35,39–42]

CLINICAL OUTCOMES IN THREE-DIMENSIONAL ENDOSCOPY FOR ENDOSCOPIC ENDONASAL TRANSSPHENOIDAL APPROACH TO THE SELLA

Several small-scale studies have been conducted using 3DE for surgery in patients with pituitary adenomas. **Table 3** illustrates their findings and middling results regarding the superiority of 3D endoscopic systems. Although some studies showed no difference in clinical outcomes between 2D and 3D visualization systems,[3,19,27] others showed superiority of 3D[15,20,34,44] or 2D.[30,42] This discrepancy might be caused by the variability in outcome measures tested, endoscope technology assessed, tumor pathologies encountered, and experience and specialty of surgeons, among other variables. Outcome measures were inconsistent between studies, but

were mainly focused on comparing the extent of resection, perioperative factors, and postoperative complications. Perioperative factors studied included hemorrhage, operative time, CSF leak rate, visual acuity, visual fields, epistaxis, hematoma in resection cavity, pneumocephalus, meningitis, need for lumbar drain, new pituitary insufficiency, and operative revision of CSF leak.[3,19,20] Postoperative complications studied included length of stay, endocrine complications, readmission rate, sinusitis, mucocele, vision loss, and pulmonary embolism.[3,15,20] With the exception of few studies,[15,27,30] no difference in clinical quantitative measures was found when comparing the 2D and 3D neuroendoscopic systems.[3,19,20,42,44] Barkhoudarian and colleagues[15] found a notable decrease in total operative time and surgical time in adenoma resection in the group using the 3D endoscope ($P = .02$ and $P = .03$). The decrease in operative time in the 3D group is consistent with other studies.[3,19] Conversely, Ogino-Nishimura and coworkers[27] found an increase in operative time in one of the cases while using a 3D endoscope. However, they believed that was caused by the extra time spent evaluating the utility of the 3D endoscope during the operation. Hajdari and colleagues[20] found that the use of 3DHD endoscopes led to a slightly better, yet statistically insignificant, resection rate of pituitary adenomas, especially ones with parasellar extension.

Subjective differences in the 2D and 3D visualization technologies were evaluated by several studies.[3,15,19,20,27,30,34,42] Depth perception could explain the "more natural feeling" and surgical comfort reported by Tabaee and colleagues[3] and Hajdari and colleagues,[20] respectively. Although the larger diameter of some 3D endoscopes is

Table 3
Clinics outcomes of 2D and 3D endoscopes for EES

Author	Number of Patients	Mean Age	Comparison	Outcome Measures	Quantitative Outcomes	Qualitative Outcomes
Brown et al,[32] 2008	12	NA	3D	Subjective operative time, other subjective measures	—	No difference in subjective operative time; enhanced depth of perception and anatomic landmark recognition
Tabaee et al,[3] 2009	13	55.5	2D vs 3D	Perioperative factors (hemorrhage, operative time, CSF leak rate, visual acuity, visual field testing, length of stay, extent of resection), questionnaire	No difference	3D enhanced depth perception, no subjective discomfort, but difficult to clean, had lack of angled scopes, and a larger scope diameter
Shah et al,[42] 2011	8	NA	3D	Intraoperative complications (image clarity, resolution of image, endoscope diameter, soiling, learning curve, depth perception	No complication	All measures were better with the 2D endoscope except for depth perception
Kari et al,[19] 2012	58	49.4	2D vs 2DHD vs 3D	Perioperative factors (estimated blood loss, operative time, CSF leak); immediate postoperative factors (length of stay, endocrine complications, and readmission rate)	No difference	3D had reduced field of view
Barkhoudarian et al,[15] 2013	160	49.7	2D vs 3D	Perioperative factors (operative time, surgical time); immediate postoperative factors (length of stay, epistaxis, SIADH/DI, sinusitis, mucocele, vision loss and pulmonary embolism), extent of resection	Decreased operative time with 3D No differences regarding other factors	With 3D, novices were quicker to learn, had less "air drilling," more accurate application of rongeurs and Kerrison punches 3D also had lower resolution images with red color saturation variation, frequent blood soiling, subjective discomfort, and higher cost

Study						
Ogino-Nishimura et al,[27] 2015	7	NA	2D vs 3D	Operative time, estimated blood loss, perioperative complications	No differences, except one case with increase operative time	3D had superior depth perception, better dissection capability, but lacked brightness, caused eye fatigue at the beginning of surgery, and soiled frequently
Nassimizadeh et al,[34] 2015	—	—	2D vs 3D vs 3DHD	—	—	3D had good depth perception, but the worst blood soiling and image quality. 3DHD was either similar or superior to 3D in all measures. 2D scopes had wider field of view with better maneuverability and ease to setup similar in all systems
Hajdari et al,[20] 2018	170	57.3	2D vs 3D vs 3DHD	Perioperative complications (epistaxis, hematoma in resection cavity, pneumocephalus, meningitis, postoperative CSF leak, lumbar drain, new pituitary insufficiency, operative revision of CSF leak, new visual deficits), tumor resection rate, postoperative improvement in visual acuity and visual fields	No differences	Improved comfort and dexterity with 3D, but better resolution and color fidelity with 2D

Abbreviations: NA, Not Applicable; SIADH, Syndrome of inappropriate secretion of antidiuretic hormone; DI, Diabetes insipidus.

sometimes cited as a concern, in a study done by Nassimizadeh and colleagues,[34] the level of maneuverability was not noticeably different among 2D, 3D standard definition, and 3DHD endoscopy. Garzaro and colleagues[45] compared nasal airflow resistance and olfactory function preoperatively and postoperatively when 3DE was used to remove sellar, parasellar, and clival pathologies, and their results were comparable with microscopic historical series. Although no direct comparative studies between 2D and 3DE in regard to olfactory function have been published, we believe that better identification of anatomic structures by 3DE allows better preservation of olfactory function.

OUR EXPERIENCE WITH THREE-DIMENSIONAL ENDOSCOPY

The development of 3DE follows in a long line of developments in rhinology and minimally invasive skull base surgery, all seeking to replicate the experience of the operating microscope within the deep recesses of the nose. The intention was to increase depth of field and surgical accuracy, and by many accounts it seems to be accomplishing this for teams that have published their results. Almost all studies indicate that tumor resection, complication rates, and visualization from 3D endoscopes are at least noninferior to 2D, with many surgeons even saying they prefer them. Yet, in the more than 10 years since they were first made available, the use of 3D for adenoma surgery remains rare and not freely adopted. In an era when more and more pituitary adenomas are being discovered and treated, this seems incongruous.

Our group operates at a high-volume pituitary tumor center of excellence, as recognized by the Pituitary Society,[46] and resects a large number of adenomas via EES every year. Our experience with 3DE via the popular "insect eye" model corroborates many of the positive aspects noted by others in the literature. Our approach typically begins with our otolaryngology colleagues, who use 2D endoscopy to perform an approach to the sphenoid sinus, wide sphenoidotomy, posterior septectomy, and nasoseptal flap harvest, if needed. The neurosurgery team then takes over and switches to 3D endoscopes for the dural opening and tumor resection. Depth of field from 3D endoscopes is substantially more accurate and allows for an appreciation of the depth of instruments within the surgical field. We use the pseudocapsular dissection technique to resect adenomas whenever possible; this relies on the separation of thin layers of tissue to allow dissection of the tumor capsule away from the neurovascular structures. Much of the 2D training for this approach relies on learning the tactile cues for cutting through these layers and massaging the plane between tumor capsule and surrounding tissues to deliver the tumor *en bloc*, and the learning curve is steep. 3DE has helped to ease this learning process for residents and fellows. The image quality of the 3D endoscope, although not in HD, is in general brighter and more color-accurate than the traditional 2D endoscopes we previously used.

We, too, recognized several of the drawbacks to 3DE. The number of specific components required for proper usage of the device is more than for 2D models, including a dedicated endoscope tower, 3D viewing screen, stereoscopic glasses, and separate power supply; none of these are cross-compatible, and if one malfunctions the whole system is often unusable. Although visual discomfort is not notable for us, viewing angles for the monitor are small and finding a position that is suitable for all operating surgeons is difficult. The smaller field of view makes resection more difficult for tumors with significant lateral extension, especially using the pseudocapsular technique; the scope has to be reoriented more frequently and can cause more intranasal trauma. The larger scope diameter sometimes requires more soft tissue dissection for exposure. For these reasons, we do not routinely use 3DE for most adenoma surgery, but reserve it for cases for which increased depth of field is advantageous (eg, significant suprasellar extension, vascular encasement, or small tumor size). We anticipate that with further development of 3DE technology, particularly with regard to the ergonomics of viewing monitors, endoscope size, and cross-compatibility with other systems, we will find it easier to use routinely. We find distinct advantages to 3DE that will be key to our practice once efficiency improves.

SUMMARY

Skull base endoscopy, in particular the EES, has revolutionized pituitary adenoma surgery. Patients around the world now have access to minimally invasive removal of tumors that are debilitating. 3DE represents the next step in trying to replicate human vision in this small, difficult to access corridor. The present experience suggests that 3DE has much to offer, but that more refinement of the technology may be necessary. Furthermore, as more is learned about the pathologies that are safely accessed via endoscope, more is learned about where 3DE can help and hinder progress. The added costs and technological hurdles of 3DE may be most appropriate for certain lesions (eg, large, adherent, suprasellar location) and not for others. Training with 2D and 3D endoscopes for pituitary adenomas during residency and fellowship will only grow in importance as their reach broadens. As the technology becomes more streamlined and widespread, we anticipate that 3DE will become the standard of care for patients with pituitary adenomas.

REFERENCES

1. Cushing H III. Partial hypophysectomy for acromegaly: with remarks on the function of the hypophysis. Ann Surg 1909;50(6):1002–17.
2. Lanzino GL, Laws ER, Feiz-Erfan I, et al. Transsphenoidal approach to lesions of the sella turcica: historical overview. Barrow quarterly, vol. 18. Phoenix (AZ): Barrow Neurological Institute; 2002.
3. Tabaee A, Anand VK, Fraser JF, et al. Three-dimensional endoscopic pituitary surgery. Neurosurgery 2009;64(5 Suppl 2):288–93 [discussion: 294–5].
4. Ahmed OH, Marcus S, Lebowitz RA, et al. Evolution in visualization for sinus and skull base surgery. Otolaryngol Clin North Am 2017;50(3):505–19.
5. Doglietto F, Prevedello DM, Jane JA Jr, et al. Brief history of endoscopic transsphenoidal surgery–from Philipp Bozzini to the First World Congress of Endoscopic Skull Base Surgery. Neurosurg Focus 2005;19(6):E3.
6. Mouton WG, Bessell JR, Maddern GJ. Looking back to the advent of modern endoscopy: 150th birthday of Maximilian Nitze. World J Surg 1998;22(12):1256–8.
7. Roth J, Singh A, Nyquist G, et al. Three-dimensional and 2-dimensional endoscopic exposure of midline cranial base targets using expanded endonasal and transcranial approaches. Neurosurgery 2009;65(6):1116–28 [discussion: 1128–30].
8. Kane KJ. The early history and development of endoscopic sinonasal surgery in Australia: 1985–2005. Aust J Otolaryngology 2018;1:7.
9. Carrau RL, Jho HD, Ko Y. Transnasal-transsphenoidal endoscopic surgery of the pituitary gland. Laryngoscope 1996;106(7):914–8.
10. Lee DD, Peris-Celda M, Butrymowicz A, et al. Quality of life changes following concurrent septoplasty and/or inferior turbinoplasty during endoscopic pituitary surgery. World Neurosurg 2017;98:303–7.
11. Rhoton AL Jr. The sellar region. Neurosurgery 2002;51(4 Suppl):S335–74.
12. Taylor DG, Jane JA, Oldfield EH. Resection of pituitary macroadenomas via the pseudocapsule along the posterior tumor margin: a cohort study and technical note. J Neurosurg 2018;128(2):422–8.
13. Seong S, Park SC, Jin Chung H, et al. Clinical comparison of 3D endoscopic sinonasal surgery

between 'insect eye' 3D and 'twin lens' 3D Endoscopes. J Rhinol 2016;23:102.
14. Banks MS, Read JCA, Allison RS, et al. Stereoscopy and the human visual system. SMPTE Motion Imaging J 2012;121(4):24–43.
15. Barkhoudarian G, Del Carmen Becerra Romero A, Laws ER. Evaluation of the 3-dimensional endoscope in transsphenoidal surgery. Neurosurgery 2013;73(1 Suppl Operative):ons74–8 [discussion ons78–9].
16. Bae SY, Korniski RJ, Shearn M, et al. 4-mm-diameter three-dimensional imaging endoscope with steerable camera for minimally invasive surgery (3-D-MARVEL). Neurophotonics 2017;4(1):011008.
17. Taffinder N, Smith SG, Huber J, et al. The effect of a second-generation 3D endoscope on the laparoscopic precision of novices and experienced surgeons. Surg Endosc 1999;13(11):1087–92.
18. Badani KK, Bhandari A, Tewari A, et al. Comparison of two-dimensional and three-dimensional suturing: is there a difference in a robotic surgery setting? J Endourol 2005;19(10):1212–5.
19. Kari E, Oyesiku NM, Dadashev V, et al. Comparison of traditional 2-dimensional endoscopic pituitary surgery with new 3-dimensional endoscopic technology: intraoperative and early postoperative factors. Int Forum Allergy Rhinol 2012;2(1):2–8.
20. Hajdari S, Kellner G, Meyer A, et al. Endoscopic endonasal surgery for removal of pituitary adenomas: a surgical case series of treatment results using different 2- and 3-dimensional visualization systems. World Neurosurg 2018;119:e80–6.
21. Jho HD, Carrau RL, Ko Y, et al. Endoscopic pituitary surgery: an early experience. Surg Neurol 1997;47(3):213–22 [discussion 222–3].
22. Snyderman CH, Fernandez-Miranda J, Gardner PA. Training in neurorhinology: the impact of case volume on the learning curve. Otolaryngol Clin North Am 2011;44(5):1223–8.
23. Byrn JC, Schluender S, Divino CM, et al. Three-dimensional imaging improves surgical performance for both novice and experienced operators using the da Vinci Robot System. Am J Surg 2007;193(4):519–22.
24. Blavier A, Gaudissart Q, Cadiere GB, et al. Comparison of learning curves and skill transfer between classical and robotic laparoscopy according to the viewing conditions: implications for training. Am J Surg 2007;194(1):115–21.
25. Pennacchietti V, Garzaro M, Grottoli S, et al. Three-dimensional endoscopic endonasal approach and outcomes in sellar lesions: a single-center experience of 104 cases. World Neurosurg 2016;89:121–5.
26. Becker H, Melzer A, Schurr MO, et al. 3-D video techniques in endoscopic surgery. Endosc Surg Allied Technol 1993;1(1):40–6.

27. Ogino-Nishimura E, Nakagawa T, Sakamoto T, et al. Efficacy of three-dimensional endoscopy in endonasal surgery. Auris Nasus Larynx 2015;42(3): 203–7.

28. Fuminari K, Hideki A, Manabu O, et al. Extended endoscopic endonasal surgery using three-dimensional endoscopy in the intra-operative MRI suite for supra-diaphragmatic ectopic pituitary adenoma. Turk Neurosurg 2015;25(3):503–7.

29. Catapano G, de Notaris M, Di Maria D, et al. The use of a three-dimensional endoscope for different skull base tumors: results of a preliminary extended endonasal surgical series. Acta Neurochir (Wien) 2016;158(8):1605–16.

30. Van Gompel JJ, Tabor MH, Youssef AS, et al. Field of view comparison between two-dimensional and three-dimensional endoscopy. Laryngoscope 2014; 124(2):387–90.

31. Chan AC, Chung SC, Yim AP, et al. Comparison of two-dimensional vs three-dimensional camera systems in laparoscopic surgery. Surg Endosc 1997; 11(5):438–40.

32. Brown SM, Tabaee A, Singh A, et al. Three-dimensional endoscopic sinus surgery: feasibility and technical aspects. Otolaryngol Head Neck Surg 2008;138(3):400–2.

33. Felisati G, Pipolo C, Maccari A, et al. Transnasal 3D endoscopic skull base surgery: questionnaire-based analysis of the learning curve in 52 procedures. Eur Arch Otorhinolaryngol 2013;270(8): 2249–53.

34. Nassimizadeh A, Muzaffar SJ, Nassimizadeh M, et al. Three-dimensional hand-to-gland combat: the future of endoscopic surgery? J Neurol Surg Rep 2015;76(2):e200–4.

35. Nassimizadeh A, Zaidi SM, Nassimizadeh M, et al. Endoscopic training-is the future three-dimensional? Laryngoscope Investig Otolaryngol 2018;3(5): 345–8.

36. Felisati G, Lenzi R, Pipolo C, et al. Endoscopic expanded endonasal approach: preliminary experience with the new 3D endoscope. Acta Otorhinolaryngol Ital 2013;33(2):102–6.

37. Beer-Furlan A, Evins AI, Rigante L, et al. Dual-port 2D and 3D endoscopy: expanding the limits of the endonasal approaches to midline skull base lesions with lateral extension. J Neurol Surg B Skull Base 2014;75(3):187–97.

38. Marcus HJ, Hughes-Hallett A, Cundy TP, et al. Comparative effectiveness of 3-dimensional vs 2-dimensional and high-definition vs standard-definition neuroendoscopy: a preclinical randomized crossover study. Neurosurgery 2014;74(4): 375–80 [discussion: 380–1].

39. Kawanishi Y, Fujimoto Y, Kumagai N, et al. Evaluation of two- and three-dimensional visualization for endoscopic endonasal surgery using a novel stereo-endoscopic system in a novice: a comparison on a dry laboratory model. Acta Neurochir (Wien) 2013; 155(9):1621–7.

40. Fraser JF, Allen B, Anand VK, et al. Three-dimensional neurostereoendoscopy: subjective and objective comparison to 2D. Minimally invasive neurosurgery. Minim Invasive Neurosurg 2009; 52(1):25–31.

41. Rampinelli V, Doglietto F, Mattavelli D, et al. Two-dimensional high definition versus three-dimensional endoscopy in endonasal skull base surgery: a comparative preclinical study. World Neurosurg 2017;105:223–31.

42. Shah RN, Leight WD, Patel MR, et al. A controlled laboratory and clinical evaluation of a three-dimensional endoscope for endonasal sinus and skull base surgery. Am J Rhinol Allergy 2011;25(3): 141–4.

43. Raheja A, Kalra R, Couldwell WT. Three-dimensional versus two-dimensional neuroendoscopy: a preclinical laboratory study. World Neurosurg 2016;92: 378–85.

44. Inoue D, Yoshimoto K, Uemura M, et al. Three-dimensional high-definition neuroendoscopic surgery: a controlled comparative laboratory study with two-dimensional endoscopy and clinical application. J Neurol Surg A Cent Eur Neurosurg 2013; 74(6):357–65.

45. Garzaro M, Pecorari G, Riva G, et al. Nasal functions in three-dimensional endoscopic skull base surgery. Ann Otol Rhinol Laryngol 2018. 3489418816723. [Epub ahead of print].

46. Casanueva FF, Barkan AL, Buchfelder M, et al. Criteria for the definition of pituitary tumor centers of excellence (PTCOE): a Pituitary Society statement. Pituitary 2017;20(5):489–98.

Management of Giant Pituitary Adenomas
Role and Outcome of the Endoscopic Endonasal Surgical Approach

Miguel Marigil Sanchez, MD, PhD[a,b,*], Claire Karekezi[a,c],
Joao Paulo Almeida[a], Aristotelis Kalyvas[a], Vitor Castro[a],
Carlos Velasquez[a,d], Fred Gentili[a]

KEYWORDS

- Endoscopic • Transsphenoidal • Giant • Pituitary • Adenomas

KEY POINTS

- EEA should be considered as the initial approach for giant adenomas with the goal of safe maximal resection and decompression of the optic apparatus.
- Lateral extension of these tumors into the middle fossa or significant anterior fossa represents a limitation of the endoscopic approach.
- The endoscopic endonasal approach maintains the same safety profile for giant adenomas in comparison with other techniques.
- Combined approaches should be considered in selected cases.

INTRODUCTION

Pituitary adenomas are the third most common type of brain tumor, representing 10% to 15% of all intracranial tumors,[1,2] with the nonfunctional gonadotroph adenoma accounting for the most frequent subtype.[3] In general, pituitary tumors can be symptomatic as a result of hyperhormonal or hypohormonal production, may display a growth pattern with mass effect on adjacent structures, or may be discovered incidentally.[1]

Nonfunctioning macroadenomas represent roughly 40% of all pituitary tumors. They may be associated with clinical symptoms arising from progressive tumor growth, leading to compression of the optic apparatus, pituitary stalk, and invasion of suprasellar and parasellar structures.[1,4-8] Giant pituitary adenomas are a subset of pituitary tumors classically characterized by their large size and increased potential to invade the parasellar and suprasellar regions, leading to visual decline, ocular movement dysfunction, and hypopituitarism.[4-10]

Surgical treatment of pituitary adenomas in general has included both microscopic and endoscopic transsphenoidal approaches. However, because of their extension beyond the sella, invasion of parasellar structures, and encasement of neurovascular structures, giant pituitary adenomas pose a significant surgical challenge.[11,12] They are associated with decreased gross total resection (GTR) rates, increased

Disclosure Statement: The authors have nothing to disclose.
[a] Division of Neurosurgery, Toronto Western Hospital, University of Toronto, Toronto, Ontario, Canada;
[b] Department of Neurosurgery, Skull Base Research Unit, Lariboisière University Hospital, 2 Rue Ambroise Paré, Paris Cedex 10 75475, France; [c] Department of Neurosurgery, Rwanda Military Hospital, Kigali, Rwanda;
[d] Department of Neurological Surgery, Hospital Universitario Marques de Valdecilla and Instituto de Investigacion Marques de Valdecilla (IDIVAL), Santander, Spain
* Corresponding author. Lariboisière University Hospital, 2 Rue Ambroise Paré, Paris Cedex 10 75475, France.
E-mail address: mmarigilsanchez@gmail.com

treatment morbidity and mortality, increased recurrence rates, and overall poorer treatment outcomes and long-term prognosis.

Giant adenomas have been treated traditionally by using transcranial (TC) or transsphenoidal microscopic approaches. Over the last 2 decades with the increasing use of endoscopic techniques, numerous case series and other reports have described and analyzed the role of the endoscopic approach in the treatment of this specific and challenging subtype of pituitary tumor.[4,5,10,13]

DEFINITION OF GIANT PITUITARY ADENOMAS

Giant pituitary adenomas have been traditionally defined as tumors measuring more than 4 cm in one diameter, although a clear definition has not been reached and there remains no consensus in the literature on the precise definition.[4–10] Initially, a classification based on the degree of suprasellar and parasellar extension was used by some investigators following the Hardy classification.[14–16] This scale scores according to the suprasellar, parasellar, and lateral or asymmetric extension: A, less than 10 mm suprasellar extension; B, 10 to 20 mm reaching the third ventricle; C, 20 to 30 mm occupying the third ventricle; D, greater than 30 mm extension beyond the foramen of Monro; and E, lateral extension.[8] Other investigators have used the size of 4 or even 3 cm in at least one of the maximal diameters to be considered as giant adenomas.[10,17–22]

Recently, some investigators have proposed different criteria for characterization of these tumors, including a maximum diameter of greater than 3 cm in all 3 axes and a tumoral volume greater than 10 cm.[9,23–25] Importantly, it has been shown that those adenomas overshooting these volumetric limits may be associated with lower rates of extent of resection and a higher predisposition for extension into the parasellar areas.[9,25] Consequently, 2 methods of calculating large tumoral volumes have been described previously.[9] The first one uses a digitized MRI scan applied with specific software. The second one, easier and without any specific requirement beyond a neuronavigated MRI scan, is named the ellipsoid shape rule, defined as half of the product of the maximal anteroposterior-lateral and craniocaudal dimensions of the tumor (ABC/2 method). This latter system allows for a straightforward and accurate estimation of the volume with an excellent correlation with the data obtained with imaging software.[9,26,27]

SURGICAL INDICATIONS

Most giant pituitary adenomas, with the possible exception of giant prolactinomas, require surgical treatment to decompress critical neural structures such as the optic nerves or chiasm and, in some cases to alleviate clinical symptoms related to brain and cavernous sinus compression. The objective of surgery is to achieve maximum decompression and resection, preserving sensitive neurovascular structures and the endocrine function.[25,28–30]

Traditionally TC approaches, such as bifrontal, pterional, or orbitozigomatic craniotomies, have been used for the treatment of giant adenomas in combination with or without a microscopic transsphenoidal (MTS) approach.[4,5,10,13] Endoscopic endonasal surgery for resection of pituitary adenomas has over the last decade become an increasingly applied and viable surgical alternative for management of pituitary adenomas. The improved visualization and wider access of the sellar and parasellar regions has resulted in good clinical outcomes and tumor removal with acceptable complication rates.[9,31–34] However, data regarding the role of endoscopic surgery for giant adenomas is still limited and mostly based on single-center retrospective studies with a small number of patients. Therefore, there is currently limited evidence-based criteria for evaluation of the applicability of this technique for giant pituitary adenomas.[9,24,25,28,35]

PREOPERATIVE PLANNING

All patients with these tumors should undergo a complete preoperative assessment including imaging with computed tomography and MRI, full endocrine panel, and ophthalmologic assessment.

SURGICAL TECHNIQUE: CONTROVERSIES, NUANCES, AND PITFALLS

A description of the endoscopic endonasal approach has been comprehensively reviewed in previous papers.[36] The endonasal transsphenoidal endoscopic resection of a pituitary adenoma involves 3 major surgical phases described here: (1) the endonasal and transsphenoidal phase, (2) the tumor resection, and (3) cranial base repair. The procedure is performed by using a 4-mm diameter of 0° and 30°.

Phase 1: Endonasal and Transsphenoidal Phase

Although there is controversy regarding the need for a middle turbinectomy, the authors routinely carry out a right middle turbinectomy, which allows for a wider corridor and exposure of the nasal and sphenoid anatomy. In giant adenomas where the risk of a postoperative cerebrospinal fluid (CSF) leak is higher, a vascularized mucosal nasoseptal flap is routinely harvested.

Next, a posterior septectomy is performed to allow for a binostril bimanual microsurgical technique. On occasion a second contralateral flap is raised. This is followed by a wide sphenoidotomy that allows full visualization of the lateral optico-carotid recesses bilaterally and from the tuberculum to the clival recess. If the tumor extends significantly anteriorly and an extended approach is a consideration, the tuberculum and planum sphenoidale are exposed. The sellar bony floor is opened laterally to the medial wall of the cavernous sinus bilaterally, superiorly to the superior intracavernous sinus and inferiorly to the inferior intracavernous sinus. Again if an extended approach is contemplated, and based on the degree of anterior extension confirmed on intraoperative neuronavigation, the tuberculum and planum may be resected. Doppler ultrasonography is used routinely to identify the parasellar carotid arteries and guide the extent of the exposure. Extended approaches are used selectively in those cases where additional bone removal would increase the extent of resection.

Phase 2: Tumor Resection

The tumor is initially internally debulked in a piecemeal fashion by using the microsurgical technique as performed in open surgery. Doppler ultrasonography is a key tool for identifying the vascular structures that may be closely adhered to the tumor. Meticulous bimanual dissection is then used to dissect the tumor from the medial walls of the cavernous sinus. If a clear plane is found this may allow in some, but not all cases, for an extracapsular dissection. Next, based on the preoperative imaging, an attempt is made to identify and dissect the tumor from the pituitary gland. If the tumor is adequately removed one observes the full descent of the diaphragm. On occasion a Valsalva maneuver may help the diaphragm descend.

Phase 3: Skull Base Repair

Although there is still no consensus about the best protocol to repair the skull base defect, a multilayer reconstruction is highly recommended. In the authors' experience, a 2-layered fascia lata graft placed intradurally and extradurally has proved to be helpful in preventing a postoperative CSF leak. This is followed by placing the pedicled nasoseptal flap(s) to cover the entire bony defect,

making sure the edges of the flap are in contact with the exposed bone to maximize their healing properties. Finally, the last layers are placed as follows: Surgicel (Ethicon), tissue glue (Tisseel, Baxter), and collagen sponge. In extended procedures a nasal Foley catheter or packing is used for 3 to 4 days to prevent graft migration. A lumbar drain is not used routinely.

SURGICAL OUTCOME

Pituitary adenoma surgery has experienced a steady evolution since its introduction by Cushing and has evolved into the classic microsurgical transsphenoidal route popularized by Hardy.[8,23,37,38]

Subsequently the improvement in endoscopic techniques, technological modifications, and the implementation of better light sources and high-definition cameras have allowed for improved visualization and excellent panoramic view of the sellar, parasellar, and suprasellar areas, leading to the increasing use of endoscopic techniques for pituitary adenomas.[39,40] Numerous groups have demonstrated the equivalency and possible superiority of endoscopic approaches over the traditional microscopic techniques for the removal of pituitary adenomas, whether in functioning or nonfunctioning lesions. Endoscopic resection has also been shown to have better visual outcomes, pituitary function preservation, and overall low complication rates attributed to the ability to achieve better suprasellar access.[31,41–43]

There is still a lack of consensus regarding the utility or benefits of the endoscopic approaches for giant adenomas, owing to the nature and extension of these tumors. Therefore, by following the PRISMA (Preferred Reporting Items for Systematic Reviews and Meta-Analysis) guidelines[44] and after performing a systematic search for randomized and nonrandomized trials, case controls, and observational studies of the endoscopic surgical treatment of giant pituitary adenomas in the Cochrane Library, MEDLINE, and EMBASE databases, 925 relevant studies were identified once duplicates were excluded.

Inclusion criteria were then applied to PICOS (participants, interventions, comparisons, outcomes, and study design) (**Table 1**) to exclude 824 studies. Case series with fewer than 10 patients or with inconsistent follow-up periods were also excluded. Those studies in which more than one surgical technique was used and where no specific data for each technique were reported were also excluded from the analysis. Giant pituitary adenomas were considered as those tumors measuring greater than 3 cm in at least one

Table 1	
Inclusion criteria applied in the systematic review of endoscopic surgery for giant adenoma	
PICOS Criteria	**Inclusion Criteria**
Participants	Patients diagnosed with giant adenomas treated surgically and with at least 1 y of postoperative follow-up
Interventions	Endoscopic endonasal surgical resection
Comparison	Comparison with other treatments was not assessed
Outcomes	Primary: extent of resection Secondary: visual improvement, postoperative complications
Study design	Observational studies, meta-analysis and systematic reviews

Abbreviation: PICOS, participants, interventions, comparisons, outcomes, and study design.

maximal diameter and/or volume greater than 10 mL, as reported in previous publications.[9,24,25] Only patients who underwent endoscopic endonasal surgery for resection of giant adenomas and had a follow-up of at least 1 year were included.

Consequently, 101 articles were assessed with a full-text review approach. Among these, 87 were finally excluded because of insufficient data, inclusion of tumors other than pituitary adenomas, and/or application of surgical techniques other than endoscopic approaches (**Fig. 1**). In total 12 studies, summarized in **Table 2**, in which a pure endoscopic approach was used as the first modality for giant adenomas, were included in this systematic review[9,15,17,18,21,24,25,28,29,45–47] (see **Fig. 1**). The combined results for primary/secondary outcomes obtained after the data extraction are summarized in **Table 3**. In total, 431 patients who underwent endoscopic

endonasal approach as the primary treatment for giant adenomas were identified.

We describe the results of this analysis regarding extent of resection, visual improvement, and surgical complications (CSF leak, postoperative hormonal dysfunction, vascular injury, and death) (see **Table 1**).

Extent of Resection

There is considerable heterogeneity in the literature regarding the extent of resection (EOR) rates for giant pituitary adenomas in different published studies that included combined microscopic approaches[4,5,13,19,48,49] and some with one single surgical technique, either endoscopic or microscopic.[9,18,24,25,28,29,35,45,50] Many series in the literature have reported low rates of tumor resection for giant pituitary adenomas despite considerable advances and improvement in surgical techniques over the last 2 decades.[4,5,9,18,24,25,28,29,35,45,46,50] The MTS approach has been adopted as the primary surgical approach in the treatment of these tumors because adequate tumor resection could be achieved with relatively minimal morbidity and mortality when compared with the classic TC approaches.[5,10,51]

The expanded endoscopic endonasal approach (EEA) allows the surgeon to safely treat complex tumors with suprasellar and parasellar extensions and cavernous sinus invasions because of the wider angle of vision provided by the endoscope, and has been associated with lower surgical risks.[9,31–33,40,52] The open TC approach has been suggested as a second-choice alternative particularly with more asymmetric tumors, and has remained a useful technique to decompress the optic apparatus and easily access the lateral extent of tumors into the middle cranial fossa.[5,10,51] Nevertheless, it requires manipulation of the optic apparatus with more difficult control of its vascular supply underlying the tumor, as the approach is based from above using a narrower trajectory. These limitations may compromise vision and have been associated with a higher risk of vascular injury and stroke as well as higher morbidity.[10,20,51,53]

Komotar and colleagues[20] conducted the only systematic review published so far addressing the surgical treatment of giant adenomas and identified 11 relevant studies (3 EEA, 6 MTS, 3 TC, and 2 combined EEA and endoscopic transventricular). In the EEA cohort, GTR in the 3 studies was achieved in 47.2% of patients and subtotal resection in the remaining 52.8%. Based on their results, they found statistically significantly higher rates of GTR in the endoscopic cohort and

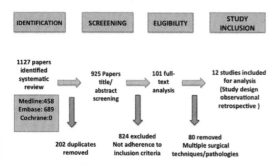

Fig. 1. Data-collection strategy.

Table 2
Studies included in the systematic review for endoscopic surgery in giant adenomas: study design, reported outcomes, and conclusions

Study, Year	Study Design and No. of Patients	No. of Patients	Primary Outcome (EOR)	Secondary Outcomes	Conclusions
Koutourousiou et al,[28] 2013	Retrospective cohort study	54	GTR: 11 patients (20%) NTR: 36 patients (67%) GTR in 6.1% of irregular tumors or lateral extension or CS invasion Knosp grade 3–4 A lower EOR rate is associated with CS invasion (Knosp grades 3–4)	Vision improvement (VA/VF): 36 patients (80%) CSF leak: 9 patients (17%) New partial hypopituitary dysfunction: 9 patients (16%) New permanent DI: 5 patients (10%) Hematoma: 2 patients (3%) Mortality: 3 patients (5%)	Goals for GA endoscopic surgery should be safe tumor resection and decompression of optic apparatus Vision improvement rate with EEA is similar to previous MTS series and the postoperative complications are less than with TC approaches The EEA is limited in tumors with middle or posterior fossa extension
Hofstetter et al,[24] 2012	Retrospective case series	20	GTR: 8 patients (40%) CS invasion and preop. volume >10 cm³ increases the likelihood of STR	VF improvement: 12 patients (86%) New panhypopituitarism: 3 patients (15%) New permanent DI: 2 patients (10%) Vascular injury (ophthalmic artery): 1 patient (5%)	Tumor volume >10 cm³ and cavernous sinus invasion is helpful to predict the likelihood of STR For GAs, EEA is associated with safer and higher rates of resection regardless of the suprasellar extension
Cusimano et al,[9] 2012	Retrospective cohort study (subgroup of 29 patients)	29	GTR: 6 patients (21%) Mean volume reduction 91%	Vision improvement (VA/VF): 24 patients (92%) (out of 26 with preoperative visual deficit) CSF leak: 1 pt (3%) New partial hypopituitarism: 9 patients (31%) New permanent DI: 2 patients (7%)	Better oncologic and endocrine outcomes for GA with EEA compared with retrospective series of MTS or TC Safer decompression and visual outcomes with EEA

(continued on next page)

Table 2
(continued)

Study, Year	Study Design and No. of Patients	No. of Patients	Primary Outcome (EOR)	Secondary Outcomes	Conclusions
Sankhla et al,[15] 2013	Retrospective cohort study	13	GTR: 8 patients (62%) STR: 4 patients (30%) PR: 1 patient (8%)	Vision improvement: 12 patients (90%) CSF leak: 4 patients (30%) New hypothalamic injury: 1 patient (8%)	Expanded EEA offers an alternative in GAs with purely midline location Better control for compression-related symptoms with EEA
Gondim et al,[18] 2014	Retrospective cohort study	50	GTR: 19 patients (38%) NTR: 9 patients (18%) STR: 22 patients (44%) The degree of resection is inversely correlated with the Knosp grade	Vision improvement: 38 patients (76%) CSF leak: 4 patients (8%) New hypopituitarism: 18 patients (47%) New permanent DI: 5 patients (10%) Mortality: 1 pt (2%)	EEA is the initial recommended approach for GA with the goal of visual decompression Preoperative Knosp grade 3 is associated with subtotal resection
Juraschka et al,[25] 2014	Retrospective cohort study	73	GTR 16 patients (24%) NTR (>90%): 11 patients (17%) STR (70%–89.9%): 24 patients (36%) PR (<70%): 15 (23%) Average EOR: 82.9% GTR is associated with Knosp and volume >10 cm³	VA improvement: 46/63 patients (73%) VF improvement: 34 patients (62%) CSF leak: 7 patients (10%) New panhypopituitarism: 4 patients (6%) Transient inappropriate secretion of ADH: 3 patients (4.1%)	The EEA approach provides reasonable EOR rates, favorable clinical outcomes, and decompression of neural structures with low complication rates Knosp grade >2 and volume >10 cm³ may decrease the likelihood of complete resection
Chabot et al,[45] 2015	Retrospective cohort study	39	GTR: 22 patients (56%) NTR: 11 patients (28%) STR: 6 patients (15%) Knosp grade is inversely associated with EOR	Vision improvement or unchanged: 39 patients (100%) CSF leak: 4 patients (10%) No postoperative hormonal deficits: 29 patients (74%) New permanent DI: 3 patients (8%)	EEA for giant pituitary adenomas is safe and efficient EOR rates are higher and complications rates are lower than in microscopic series

Study	Study type	N	Resection	Outcomes/complications	Conclusions
Landeiro et al,[29] 2015	Retrospective case series	35	GTR: 21 patients (55%)	VF improvement: 17 patients (74%) VA improvement: 20 patients (80%) Visual worsening: 2 patients (6%) CSF leak: 1 patient (3%) Vascular injury (ICA): 1 patient (3%) New hormonal deficit: 0 patients (0%) Transient DI: 9 patients (26%)	EEA provides good control rates and optic apparatus decompression of GNFPA It is recommended to closely follow-up with surveillance and to reserve the adjuvant therapy for progressive growth or symptoms
Yildirim et al,[47] 2016	Retrospective case series	20	GTR: 14 patients (70%) STR: 6 patients (30%)	CFS leak: 1 patient (5%) New panhypopituitarism: 3 patients (15%) New permanent DI: 2 patients (10%)	GA treated with EEA can obtain good visual outcomes with low risk for pituitary injury
Constantino et al,[17] 2016	Retrospective cohort study	28	GTR: 4 patients (14%) NTR: 3 patients (11%) STR: 11 patients (39%) PR: 10 patients (36%)	Vision improvement: 9 patients (32.1%) CSF leak: 5 patients (17.8%) New permanent DI: 1 patient (4%) Mortality: 2 patients (7%)	EEA for GA offers higher rates of surgical decompression in neurovascular structures and fewer short- and long-term complications
Kuo et al,[21] 2016	Retrospective cohort study	38	GTR: 8 patients (21%) STR: 30 patients (79%)	Vision improvement: 27 patients (71.1%) CSF leak: 0 patients (0%) New partial anterior pituitary deficiency: 10 patients (26%) New permanent DI: 1 patient (3%) Hematoma: 3 patients (9%) Vascular injury (ICA): 1 patient (3%)	EEA is a safe and effective surgical approach for GAs
Yano et al,[46] 2017	Retrospective cohort study	32	NTR (<10% residual): 16 patients (47%) PR: 18 patients (53%) Middle cranial extension and/or lobular configuration is associated with less EOR	VF improvement: 23/25 patients (92%) CSF leak: 2 patients (5.9%) New anterior pituitary deficiency: 4 patients (11.8%) New permanent DI: 7 patients (20.6%)	EEA allows for safer removal of GAs regardless of the size or configuration of the suprasellar component Good rates of visual preservation and improvement in VF impairment

Abbreviations: CS, cavernous sinus; CSF, cerebrospinal fluid; DI, diabetes insipidus; EEA, expanded endoscopic endonasal approach; EOR, extent of resection; GA, giant adenoma; GNFPA, giant nonfunctioning pituitary adenoma; GTR, gross total resection; ICA, internal carotid artery; MTS, microscopic transsphenoidal; NTR, near total resection (>90%); PR, partial resection; STR, subtotal resection (<90%); TC, transcranial approach; VA, visual acuity; VF, visual fields.

Table 3
Overall primary and secondary outcomes of endoscopic surgery in GA

Outcome	n (%)
Primary outcome	
1. EOR[a]	
GTR	137 (34.0)
STR/PR	192 (48.0)
NTR	70 (18)
Secondary outcomes	
1. Visual function outcome	
Visual improvement[b]	(71–97.4)
2. Postoperative Complications	
CSF leak	38 (8.8)
New permanent DI and/or anterior hypophyseal deficit	90 (20.8)
Ischemic/arterial injuries[c]	6 (0.01)
Intracranial hematoma[d]	4 (0.01)
Hydrocephalus	3 (0.01)
Mortality	6 (1.39)
Total of patients	431 (100)

Pooled data from the 12 studies included in the systematic review.

Abbreviations: CSF, cerebrospinal fluid; DI, diabetes insipidus; EOR, extent of resection; GA, giant adenoma; GTR, gross total resection; NTR, near total resection (>90%); PR, partial resection; STR, subtotal resection (<90%); VA, visual acuity; VF, visual fields.

[a] The extent of resection was not reported for 32 patients by Yano and colleagues,[46] so only 399 had available data for total percentages.

[b] Improvement in either visual acuity or in visual field preoperative deficit.

[c] Two internal carotid artery and 1 ophthalmic artery pseudoaneurysm treated with an endovascular approach, and 3 strokes attributable to perforator branch injuries.

[d] Three needed surgical treatment; 1 death.

transsphenoidal cohort than in the open cohort, and a higher rate of GTR in the EEA than in the MTS groups. Noticeably, this systematic review includes only one purely endoscopic cohort for 43 giant adenomas. However, despite the superiority in favor of endoscopic techniques, the major limitation of this review is the paucity of endoscopic studies and the heterogeneity of the techniques involved in all selected series, with no clear comparison outcomes available.

Regarding MTS approaches, Sinha and Sharma[16] published one of the biggest series of microscopic sublabial technique for tumors greater than 4 cm. They included 250 patients divided into 4 groups according to the Hardy classification. They were able to achieve near total resection (NTR) in 88% for group A, 76% for group B, and

68% and 55% for groups C and D, respectively. These investigators concluded that this technique might be beneficial for tumors with grades A and B according to the Hardy classification. Similarly, Saito and colleagues[14] published a cohort of 100 patients with multiple surgeries: 89 underwent single MTS and 14 underwent staged procedures, with 7 undergoing TC combined with MTS approach. The overall GTR was reported to be 63.2% but analysis of the EOR in each subgroup was not feasible.

In the authors' systematic review, 12 papers addressing specifically the EOR as a primary outcome through a purely EEA approach were identified. In 2 of the biggest retrospective series by Juraschka and colleagues,[25] which included 73 patients, and Koutourousiou and colleagues[28] including 54 patients, wherein all patients underwent an expanded transplanum endoscopic approach, GTR was reported to be 24.2% with NTR of 16.7% by the Juraschka group[25] and 20.4% GTR with 66.7% NTR by Koutourousiou and colleagues.[28] In a previous retrospective cohort, Cusimano and colleagues,[9] who performed an EEA for 29 patients among 72 patients who presented with giant adenoma (defined according to the volumetric criteria >10 cm³), GTR was reported to be 21%. Similarly, Gondim and colleagues,[18] in a retrospective cohort of 50 patients with pituitary adenomas defined by a maximal diameter greater than 4 cm who underwent EEA, GTR was achieved in 38%. Interestingly, Sankhla and colleagues,[15] who performed an expanded transplanum-transtuberculum EEA in 13 patients with giant pituitary adenomas, achieved an even higher GTR of 61.5%. More recently, Yildrim and colleagues,[47] in a large series of 485 surgically treated pituitary adenomas, defined 20 of these as giant pituitary adenoma (>4 cm) treated by a pure EEA. According to the investigators, GTR was achieved in 14 of 20 patients in these series (70%); this relatively higher rate of EOR was attributed to the ability of the endoscope to visualize and decompress from below with an improved illumination of the surgical field facilitating access to the tumors despite the suprasellar/parasellar invasion.

All of these reports confirm the role of safe maximal resection obtained through a purely endoscopic approach to giant adenomas.

Comparison of Endoscopic Technique with Other Techniques: Improved Extent of Resection with Surgical Limitations

Overall, analysis of all the data from the systematic review produced a GTR rate of 31.55% in a total of

431 patients who underwent EEA. These results are similar to those reported by Komotar and colleagues,[20] although the authors' review includes a considerably larger number of studies, the analysis of which suggests that the rates of GTR for endoscopic techniques are currently in the range of 32% with a 45.5% rate of subtotal resection. The better results obtained in the MTS series performed by Karki and colleagues[19] may be related to more favorable tumor selection in a smaller cohort of 123 patients in whom only 44 tumors were identified as giant as opposed to the more aggressive profile of those tumors included in the current endoscopic series. As with all retrospective series, this may reflect a selection bias in the same way that one of the endoscopic cohort describes a GTR rate close to 70% in a smaller sample of patients.[47] The authors consider that the endoscopic technique should be evaluated by its ability to safely decompress sellar and suprasellar structures and not only the extent of tumor resection.

Lateral Tumoral Configuration as a Contraindication for Endoscopic Approaches

Koutourousiou and colleagues[28] found that primary giant pituitary adenomas had a better surgical outcome compared with previously available surgical outcomes, and identified some surgical limitations for endoscopy applied in giant adenomas.[28] In general, the more complex tumor configuration, defined as extension in the coronal plane into the cavernous sinus or temporal fossa, the lower the resection rate attained. Hence, more than 90% of round giant pituitary adenomas were resected in 93% of the cases, with GTR of 46.7%, in their study. On the other hand, GTR for irregular tumor configuration occurred in only 6.1%. Although the resection rates depend on multivariate parameters, significant intracranial tumor extension such as subfrontal or temporal location has been associated with lower rates of GTR. In these cases an open TC approach is favored.[16,20,50]

Visual Outcome

In their systematic review, Komotar and colleagues[20] reported better visual outcomes and a lower complication profile in favor of endoscopic endonasal techniques. Nevertheless, it is important to clarify that only one purely endoscopic study was included in the final evaluation, and some studies included a combination of surgical techniques.[20] In this review the rate of visual improvement was reported as 91.1% (range 71% to 97.4%) in the endoscopy series compared with 40.0% and 34.8% for open and microscopic series, respectively. Although this is so far the most recent comprehensive report of giant adenoma surgical series, some of the limitations linked to the heterogeneity of existing data prevent surgeons from generalizing these results in favor of one technique.

Saito and colleagues[14] reported an overall improved visual acuity and visual field tests in 76% and 72%, respectively, in 100 patients treated with the microscopic technique, but it is important to clarify that 14 of 100 patients underwent a staged TC approach, which may explain the higher rate of visual recovery compared with other series. On the other hand, Sinha and Sharma,[16] analyzing surgical outcomes for giant adenomas that underwent TC or MTS approaches, report a moderate rate of visual improvement on the order of 53% overall.[16] The investigators acknowledge that the MTS approach may be more beneficial for those tumors without asymmetric extension, with poorer visual outcomes in those patients who required combined open and transsphenoidal procedures in Hardy grades C and D.

Finally, Mortini and colleagues[10] compared the results of 111 surgeries performed in 95 patients, 85 described as a combined microscopic and endoscopically-assisted transsphenoidal and 26 as an open technique. They showed an overall visual recovery rate in the range of 74.7%. However, the study analyzed the impact of both TC and transsphenoidal techniques on visual outcomes without differentiating surgical modalities, and 16 patients from both subgroups received multiple combined approaches in the first 6 months of the study.

Taking into account the articles included in the analysis presented in **Table 3**, one finds that endoscopic endonasal approaches provide a range of visual improvement (visual acuity and/or visual field) between 71.1% and 92% in the 12 studies evaluated from a total of 431 patients, although the total number of patients with preoperative deficits is not included in all studies. There is one article in which a rate of improvement is reported as 32.1%; however, only 42% of the patients were reported with visual deficits preoperatively and visual fields were not tested.[17] Taking into account all of the studies, only in 9 patients was visual deterioration reported.

In conclusion, the results of the systematic review reported herein are in line with reports by other investigators[20] in that the degree of visual improvement is significant with the endoscopic approach regardless of the size of the adenoma.

SURGICAL COMPLICATIONS

A CSF leak rate of 8.81% (38 patients) and observed in a total of 431 patients included in this review. This figure may be overestimated, as the vascularized nasoseptal flap reconstruction technique was introduced later on in some endoscopic series included herein. However, a different analysis establishing such a comparison is not possible with the existing data.

Regarding endocrinologic complications, a total of 90 (20.88%) patients developed a new permanent endocrinologic deficit related either to an anterior hypophyseal deficit or diabetes insipidus (DI). Ischemic injury was described in 6 patients with 3 of them suffering a pseudoaneurysm in the carotid/ophthalmic artery that required endovascular treatment. A mortality rate related to surgery of 1.39% (6 patients) was found in this endoscopic series.

In contrast, Karki and colleagues,[19] in their series of 123 patients who underwent MTS surgery, reported a CSF rate as high as 18.6% (23 patients) and new endocrinologic deficit rate of 29.2% (36 patients).

In the early series comparing the advantages and disadvantages of endoscopic endonasal surgery against the standard MTS approach, the endoscopic technique showed its relevance as a less invasive tool, obtaining better clinical and endocrinological outcomes compared with microscopic techniques for pituitary adenomas. Overall, EOR and visual outcomes have been proved to be superior with the endoscopic endonasal approaches, with CSF leak rates lower than 5% after the advent and implementation of the vascularized nasoseptal flap.[31,32,54,55]

When the data available for complications in endoscopic pituitary surgery are extrapolate, one can confirm that the rate of CSF leak and new pituitary insufficiency is higher for giant adenomas as expected in these more aggressive tumors, but is still lower than with MTS or TC techniques for pituitary macroadenomas, which has been reported to be as high as 55%.[20,56]

Although a direct comparison is not possible between this systematic review and the information available in the literature for open/microscopic techniques, the endoscopic endonasal approach seems to maintain the same profile of safety applied for giant adenomas in comparison with other techniques. In the authors' opinion, the endoscopic endonasal technique should be considered the first alternative in the surgical armamentarium when dealing with these tumors, based on its safety profile in alleviating symptoms related to tumor compression and maximizing tumor resection.

SUMMARY

Giant pituitary adenomas remain a significant surgical challenge regardless of the approach or technique used, and a volume-based threshold may be a better predictor of EOR and complications.

The endoscopic approach can provide equivalent and possibly better outcomes than the standard microsurgical approach in terms of better EOR, visual improvement, and fewer complications. The markedly improved visualization and wider access to sellar/parasellar and suprasellar structures, and less invasive nature, make it the preferred technique for the removal of most giant pituitary adenomas.

Open craniotomy or combined approaches, especially in those lesions with lateral extension, may be required. However, giant pituitary adenomas often require a multimodality approach with adjuvant radiation and/or medical therapy to effect long-term control.

REFERENCES

1. Aflorei ED, Korbonits M. Epidemiology and etiopathogenesis of pituitary adenomas. J Neurooncol 2014;117:379–94.
2. Ezzat S, Asa SL, Couldwell WT, et al. The prevalence of pituitary adenomas: a systematic review. Cancer 2004;101:613–9.
3. Mete O, Cintosun A, Pressman I, et al. Epidemiology and biomarker profile of pituitary adenohypophysial tumors. Mod Pathol 2018;31(6):900–9.
4. Garibi J, Pomposo I, Villar G, et al. Giant pituitary adenomas: clinical characteristics and surgical results. Br J Neurosurg 2002;16:133–9.
5. Goel A, Nadkarni T, Muzumdar D, et al. Giant pituitary tumors: a study based on surgical treatment of 118 cases. Surg Neurol 2004;61:436–45 [discussion: 445–6].
6. Jane JA Jr, Laws ER Jr. The surgical management of pituitary adenomas in a series of 3,093 patients. J Am Coll Surg 2001;193:651–9.
7. Laws ER, Jane JA Jr. Neurosurgical approach to treating pituitary adenomas. Growth Horm IGF Res 2005;15(Suppl A):S36–41.
8. Mohr G, Hardy J, Comtois R, et al. Surgical management of giant pituitary adenomas. Can J Neurol Sci 1990;17:62–6.
9. Cusimano MD, Kan P, Nassiri F, et al. Outcomes of surgically treated giant pituitary tumours. Can J Neurol Sci 2012;39:446–57.
10. Mortini P, Barzaghi R, Losa M, et al. Surgical treatment of giant pituitary adenomas: strategies and results in a series of 95 consecutive patients. Neurosurgery 2007; 60:993–1002 [discussion: 1003–4].

11. Buchfelder M. Management of aggressive pituitary adenomas: current treatment strategies. Pituitary 2009;12:256–60.

12. Cappabianca P, Cavallo LM, Esposito F, et al. Extended endoscopic endonasal approach to the midline skull base: the evolving role of transsphenoidal surgery. Adv Tech Stand Neurosurg 2008;33: 151–99.

13. de Paiva Neto MA, Vandergrift A, Fatemi N, et al. Endonasal transsphenoidal surgery and multimodality treatment for giant pituitary adenomas. Clin Endocrinol (Oxf) 2010;72:512–9.

14. Saito K, Kuwayama A, Yamamoto N, et al. The transsphenoidal removal of nonfunctioning pituitary adenomas with suprasellar extensions: the open sella method and intentionally staged operation. Neurosurgery 1995;36:668–75 [discussion: 675–6].

15. Sankhla SK, Jayashankar N, Khan GM. Surgical management of selected pituitary macroadenomas using extended endoscopic endonasal transsphenoidal approach: early experience. Neurol India 2013;61:122–30.

16. Sinha S, Sharma BS. Giant pituitary adenomas—an enigma revisited. Microsurgical treatment strategies and outcome in a series of 250 patients. Br J Neurosurg 2010;24:31–9.

17. Constantino ER, Leal R, Ferreira CC, et al. Surgical outcomes of the endoscopic endonasal transsphenoidal approach for large and giant pituitary adenomas: institutional experience with special attention to approach-related complications. Arq Neuropsiquiatr 2016;74:388–95.

18. Gondim JA, Almeida JP, Albuquerque LA, et al. Giant pituitary adenomas: surgical outcomes of 50 cases operated on by the endonasal endoscopic approach. World Neurosurg 2014;82:e281–90.

19. Karki M, Sun J, Yadav CP, et al. Large and giant pituitary adenoma resection by microscopic transsphenoidal surgery: Surgical outcomes and complications in 123 consecutive patients. J Clin Neurosci 2017;44:310–4.

20. Komotar RJ, Starke RM, Raper DM, et al. Endoscopic endonasal compared with microscopic transsphenoidal and open transcranial resection of giant pituitary adenomas. Pituitary 2012;15:150–9.

21. Kuo CH, Yen YS, Wu JC, et al. Primary endoscopic transnasal transsphenoidal surgery for giant pituitary adenoma. World Neurosurg 2016;91:121–8.

22. Sanai N, Quinones-Hinojosa A, Narvid J, et al. Safety and efficacy of the direct endonasal transsphenoidal approach for challenging sellar tumors. J Neurooncol 2008;87:317–25.

23. Boggan JE, Tyrrell JB, Wilson CB. Transsphenoidal microsurgical management of Cushing's disease. Report of 100 cases. J Neurosurg 1983;59:195–200.

24. Hofstetter CP, Nanaszko MJ, Mubita LL, et al. Volumetric classification of pituitary macroadenomas predicts outcome and morbidity following endoscopic endonasal transsphenoidal surgery. Pituitary 2012;15:450–63.

25. Juraschka K, Khan OH, Godoy BL, et al. Endoscopic endonasal transsphenoidal approach to large and giant pituitary adenomas: institutional experience and predictors of extent of resection. J Neurosurg 2014;121:75–83.

26. Vieira JO Jr, Cukiert A, Liberman B. Evaluation of magnetic resonance imaging criteria for cavernous sinus invasion in patients with pituitary adenomas: logistic regression analysis and correlation with surgical findings. Surg Neurol 2006;65:130–5 [discussion: 135].

27. Yu YL, Lee MS, Juan CJ, et al. Calculating the tumor volume of acoustic neuromas: comparison of ABC/2 formula with planimetry method. Clin Neurol Neurosurg 2013;115:1371–4.

28. Koutourousiou M, Gardner PA, Fernandez-Miranda JC, et al. Endoscopic endonasal surgery for giant pituitary adenomas: advantages and limitations. J Neurosurg 2013;118:621–31.

29. Landeiro JA, Fonseca EO, Monnerat AL, et al. Nonfunctioning giant pituitary adenomas: invasiveness and recurrence. Surg Neurol Int 2015;6:179.

30. Mastronardi L, Guiducci A, Spera C, et al. Ki-67 labelling index and invasiveness among anterior pituitary adenomas: analysis of 103 cases using the MIB-1 monoclonal antibody. J Clin Pathol 1999;52: 107–11.

31. Dehdashti AR, Ganna A, Karabatsou K, et al. Pure endoscopic endonasal approach for pituitary adenomas: early surgical results in 200 patients and comparison with previous microsurgical series. Neurosurgery 2008;62:1006–15 [discussion: 1015–7].

32. Di Maio S, Cavallo LM, Esposito F, et al. Extended endoscopic endonasal approach for selected pituitary adenomas: early experience. J Neurosurg 2011;114:345–53.

33. Kassam A, Snyderman CH, Mintz A, et al. Expanded endonasal approach: the rostrocaudal axis. Part I. Crista galli to the sella turcica. Neurosurg Focus 2005;19:E3.

34. Kassam A, Snyderman CH, Mintz A, et al. Expanded endonasal approach: the rostrocaudal axis. Part II. Posterior clinoids to the foramen magnum. Neurosurg Focus 2005;19:E4.

35. Nishioka H, Hara T, Nagata Y, et al. Inherent tumor characteristics that limit effective and safe resection of giant nonfunctioning pituitary adenomas. World Neurosurg 2017;106:645–52.

36. Cappabianca P, Cavallo LM, de Divitiis O, et al. Endoscopic endonasal extended approaches for the management of large pituitary adenomas. Neurosurg Clin N Am 2015;26:323–31.

37. Comtois R, Beauregard H, Somma M, et al. The clinical and endocrine outcome to trans-sphenoidal

microsurgery of nonsecreting pituitary adenomas. Cancer 1991;68:860–6.

38. Hardy J. Surgery of the pituitary gland, using the trans-sphenoidal approach. Comparative study of 2 technical methods. Union Med Can 1967;96: 702–12 [in French].

39. Gamea A, Fathi M, el-Guindy A. The use of the rigid endoscope in trans-sphenoidal pituitary surgery. J Laryngol Otol 1994;108:19–22.

40. Jankowski R, Auque J, Simon C, et al. Endoscopic pituitary tumor surgery. Laryngoscope 1992;102: 198–202.

41. Cappabianca P, Cavallo LM, Colao A, et al. Endoscopic endonasal transsphenoidal approach: outcome analysis of 100 consecutive procedures. Minim Invasive Neurosurg 2002;45:193–200.

42. Frank G, Pasquini E, Farneti G, et al. The endoscopic versus the traditional approach in pituitary surgery. Neuroendocrinology 2006;83:240–8.

43. Jho HD. Endoscopic transsphenoidal surgery. J Neurooncol 2001;54:187–95.

44. Moher D, Liberati A, Tetzlaff J, et al. Preferred reporting items for systematic reviews and meta-analyses: the PRISMA statement. Ann Intern Med 2009;151: 264–9. w264.

45. Chabot JD, Chakraborty S, Imbarrato G, et al. Evaluation of outcomes after endoscopic endonasal surgery for large and giant pituitary macroadenoma: a retrospective review of 39 consecutive patients. World Neurosurg 2015;84:978–88.

46. Yano S, Hide T, Shinojima N. Efficacy and complications of endoscopic skull base surgery for giant pituitary adenomas. World Neurosurg 2017;99:533–42.

47. Yildirim AE, Sahinoglu M, Ekici I, et al. Nonfunctioning pituitary adenomas are really clinically nonfunctioning? Clinical and endocrinological symptoms and outcomes with endoscopic endonasal treatment. World Neurosurg 2016;85:185–92.

48. Messerer M, De Battista JC, Raverot G, et al. Evidence of improved surgical outcome following endoscopy for nonfunctioning pituitary adenoma removal. Neurosurg Focus 2011;30:E11.

49. Musluman AM, Cansever T, Yilmaz A, et al. Surgical results of large and giant pituitary adenomas with special consideration of ophthalmologic outcomes. World Neurosurg 2011;76:141–8 [discussion: 63–6].

50. Guo F, Song L, Bai J, et al. Successful treatment for giant pituitary adenomas through diverse transcranial approaches in a series of 15 consecutive patients. Clin Neurol Neurosurg 2012;114: 885–90.

51. Alleyne CH Jr, Barrow DL, Oyesiku NM. Combined transsphenoidal and pterional craniotomy approach to giant pituitary tumors. Surg Neurol 2002;57: 380–90 [discussion: 390].

52. Jho HD, Carrau RL, Ko Y, et al. Endoscopic pituitary surgery: an early experience. Surg Neurol 1997;47: 213–22 [discussion: 222–3].

53. Pratheesh R, Rajaratnam S, Prabhu K, et al. The current role of transcranial surgery in the management of pituitary adenomas. Pituitary 2013;16:419–34.

54. Kassam AB, Thomas A, Carrau RL, et al. Endoscopic reconstruction of the cranial base using a pedicled nasoseptal flap. Neurosurgery 2008;63: ONS44–52 [discussion ONS52–3].

55. O'Malley BW Jr, Grady MS, Gabel BC, et al. Comparison of endoscopic and microscopic removal of pituitary adenomas: single-surgeon experience and the learning curve. Neurosurg Focus 2008;25:E10.

56. Linsler S, Senger S, Hero-Gross R, et al. The endoscopic surgical resection of intrasellar lesions conserves the hormonal function: a negative correlation to the microsurgical technique. J Neurosurg Sci 2018. [Epub ahead of print].

Management of Pituitary Adenomas Invading the Cavernous Sinus

Martin Rutkowski, MD*, Gabriel Zada, MD, MS

KEYWORDS

- Pituitary adenomas • Cavernous sinus • Invasion • Surgery • Radiosurgery • Knosp • Endoscope

KEY POINTS

- The cavernous sinuses are complex dural venous sinuses that house important neurovascular structures, including cranial nerves and the cavernous internal carotid artery, which often preclude full surgical access for tumor resection.
- Neuro-imaging and anatomic grading scales to determine extent of cavernous invasion and subsequent surgical visualization have corroborated that more invasive tumors are less likely to undergo gross total resection and biochemical remission.
- Endoscopic approaches are increasingly favored over microsurgical techniques due to superior visualization, panoramic views, improved maneuverability of instruments, and implementation of angled endoscopes to facilitate greater extent of resection.
- The addition of direct transcavernous approaches has yielded even greater degrees of resection, and may offer incremental increases in biochemical remission for functional, invasive adenomas.
- Radiosurgery is a powerful adjuvant therapy for residual, recurrent, and/or inaccessible cavernous sinus disease that provides excellent tumor control rates and favorable risk-benefit ratios for the achievement of biochemical remission with minimal endocrine morbidity.

INTRODUCTION

Pituitary adenomas (PA) invasion into the cavernous sinus occurs in a substantial proportion of patients, variably quoted as 6% to 43% in large surgical series in the literature.[1–9] In addition to the increased surgical challenge of obtaining gross total resection, residual and often inaccessible disease within the cavernous sinus necessitates multimodality approaches that use medical and radiation-based therapies to achieve tumor control and biochemical remission, in particular with patients harboring functional PA subtypes with ongoing hormonal hypersecretion.

In the following review, we examine the role that cavernous sinus invasion plays in the management of functional and nonfunctional PAs. We review the unique anatomy of the cavernous sinus, neuro-imaging and anatomic methods to categorize invasion, the role of surgical resection with and without expanded approaches, and the emerging array of adjuvant radiotherapy-based options for residual or progressive cavernous sinus disease.

CAVERNOUS SINUS ANATOMY

The cavernous sinuses are complex anatomic structures that are inherently challenging to operate in, owing to their multilayered dural anatomy, venous inflow and outflow, and intricate neurovascular contents. They are potential dural spaces comprised of trabeculated venous channels formed by separation of the periosteal and meningeal layers of dura (**Fig. 1**).

Disclosure: The authors have nothing to disclose.
Department of Neurosurgery, Keck School of Medicine, University of Southern California, 1300 North State Street, Suite 3300, Los Angeles, CA 90033, USA
* Corresponding author.
E-mail address: Martin.Rutkowski@med.usc.edu

Neurosurg Clin N Am 30 (2019) 445–455
https://doi.org/10.1016/j.nec.2019.05.005
1042-3680/19/© 2019 Elsevier Inc. All rights reserved.

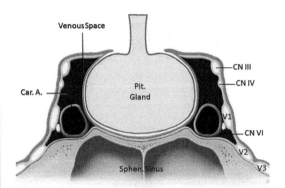

Fig. 1. Coronal representation of the cavernous sinuses surrounding the pituitary gland, with special attention to the dural layers. All but the medial wall are comprised of a periosteal (*green*) and meningeal (*orange*) layer, which split to form the potential venous space of the sinus itself. Within the lateral wall, the inner periosteal layer splits and is continuous with the epineurium of the cranial nerves, and thus houses the oculomotor nerve, trochlear nerve, ophthalmic division of the trigeminal nerve, and maxillary division of the trigeminal nerve, with the abducens nerve traveling within the cavernous sinus just lateral to the cavernous ICA. The superior wall of the cavernous sinus is continuous medially with the diaphragma sella, which has a variably sized opening that transmits the infundibulum toward the hypothalamus. (*Reprinted from* Journal of Clinical Neuroscience Volume 17, Issue 6, Alvaro Campero, Agustin Campero, Carolina Martins, Alexandre Yasuda, Albert L. Rhoton Jr., Surgical anatomy of the dural walls of the cavernous sinus, pages 746–750, Copyright 2010, with permission from Elsevier.)

Although the medial wall that abuts the pituitary gland is comprised of a single layer of meningeal dura, the lateral wall contains both layers.[10] Within the lateral wall, the oculomotor nerve travels near the cavernous sinus roof in a small cerebrospinal fluid (CSF)-filled arachnoid sleeve known as the oculomotor cistern[11] before exiting through the superior orbital fissure. Moving inferiorly, the trochlear nerve and ophthalmic (V1) and maxillary (V2) divisions of the trigeminal nerve travel within the inner periosteal layer of the lateral wall, and the abducens nerve courses through the cavernous sinus just lateral to the cavernous segment of the internal carotid artery (ICA).

The cavernous ICA gives off the meningohypophyseal trunk posteriorly to supply the inferior pituitary gland and clival/tentorial dura, and the inferolateral trunk ventrally, which variably branches to provide blood supply to the oculomotor, trochlear, abducens nerves, and the gasserian ganglion.[12] As it emerges from the cavernous sinus roof and transitions into the clinoidal segment, the ICA is tethered by the proximal dural ring,

which is continuous with the roof of the cavernous sinus, then passes through the distal dural ring, which is continuous with the falciform ligament and the dura lining the superiomedial anterior clinoid process.[13]

Superiorly, the roof of the cavernous sinus contains both layers of dura that meet and are continuous with the diaphragma sella, the dural covering comprised of both layers, which covers the pituitary gland except for an opening at its center through which the infundibulum travels to reach the median eminence of the hypothalamus.[14] Variability in the size of this opening, sphenoid bony anatomy, and the single dural layer of the medial wall of the cavernous sinuses have been postulated as reasons for variable suprasellar and lateral invasion of PAs.[1,10,14,15]

The highly complex anatomy of the cavernous sinus can make complete removal of invasive PAs technically challenging. Invasive PAs are also known to alter the position of the normal cavernous ICA, further complicating efforts at surgical extirpation.[16,17] Efforts to delineate the extent of cavernous sinus invasion with sophisticated preoperative neuro-imaging studies are mandatory in any preoperative surgical planning.

CATEGORIZATION OF PITUITARY ADENOMA INVASION

In an attempt to categorize PA invasion into the cavernous sinus on MRI, Knosp and colleagues[7] developed the Knosp-Steiner classification (**Fig. 2**). The authors examined 25 patients, 12 of whom harbored nonfunctional PAs and 13 with functional PAs. Knosp grades 0 to 4 were assigned based on preoperative coronal MRI and the relationship of PAs to the intercarotid line, an imaginary line drawn through the midpoint of the cavernous and supracavernous ICA segments. Grade 0 PAs do not encroach on the cavernous sinus, grade 1 PAs abut but do not traverse the intercarotid line, and grade 2 tumors traverse the intercarotid line but do not pass a line tangential to the lateral borders of the cavernous and supracavernous ICA segments. In the original Knosp study,[7] no patients with a grade 0 or 1 PA showed evidence of cavernous sinus invasion intraoperatively, whereas 7 of 8 patients with grade 2 tumors showed evidence of gross invasion during surgical resection. Knosp grade 3 PAs extended past the tangential line across the lateral border, and grade 4 tumors are classified as having circumferential ICA encasement. All grade 3 and 4 PAs (11 patients) demonstrated cavernous sinus invasion intraoperatively. Subsequent studies[18–20] assessing cavernous sinus invasion and surgical

Knosp Grade

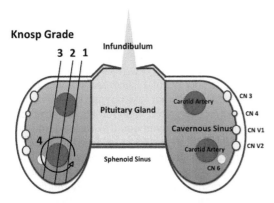

Fig. 2. The Knosp-Steiner classification scheme uses 3 grades to describe progressive cavernous sinus involvement and invasion of PAs. Grade 1 PAs abut but do not traverse the intercarotid line, grade 2 PAs traverse the intercarotid line but do not pass a line tangential to the lateral borders of the cavernous and supracavernous ICA segments, grade 3 PAs extend past the tangential line across the lateral border, and grade 4 PAs encase the ICA circumferentially. An update in 2015 established grade 3a and 3b subtypes, defined respectively as invasion beyond the lateral tangential line between ICA segments (superior compartment), and invasion below the cavernous segment and beyond the lateral tangent (inferior compartment).

outcomes based on tumor encasement of the cavernous ICA segment corroborated the results of Knosp and colleagues.

In 2015, Knosp[9] introduced an update to their original grading system of invasion, establishing the subtypes of grade 3a and 3b PAs, defined respectively as invasion beyond the lateral tangential line between ICA segments (superior compartment), and invasion below the cavernous segment and beyond the lateral tangent (inferior compartment).[9] They studied 137 PAs that were at least grade 1 and determined rates for extent of resection and biochemical remission in functioning PAs when subgrouped by Knosp grade. Importantly, they established a linear correlation between increased cavernous sinus invasion scores and decreased rates of gross total resection and biochemical remission.[9] Notably, when compared with previous data with microscopic techniques, they showed lesser discrimination of cavernous sinus invasion with microscopic examination of the medial wall compared with more modern endoscopic techniques,[9] suggesting improved visualization with the endoscope.

The Hardy classification primarily categorizes PAs according to the degree of sellar remodeling and extrasellar extension, and was developed using radiographs and encephalograms.[21–23] The Hardy classification is based on a grade of 0 to 4

for sellar invasion and A to D for suprasellar extension, with E reserved for cavernous sinus invasion. Given the inferior resolution of non-MRI-based imaging and the lack of fine characterization of cavernous sinus invasion, the Knosp score offers a more nuanced view of invasion, and may be associated with higher interrater reliability.[22,24]

EVOLVING PARADIGMS IN MICROSCOPIC AND ENDOSCOPIC APPROACHES

With increasing acceptance and use of the endoscope to facilitate PA resection, recent studies have highlighted an emerging role for endoscopy in invasive tumors, including improved visualization, access, and maneuverability when resecting PAs. Although head-to-head comparisons of overall surgical outcomes following endoscopic versus microscopic PA resections suggest further study is needed to establish superiority,[25–29] endoscopic approaches seem to offer greater extent of resection for large and invasive tumors,[20,30–38] including some series specifically addressing functional PAs and rates of biochemical remission.[39–41]

Furthermore, the endoscope may have importance as an aid to traditional microscopic techniques; McLaughlin and colleagues[42] found that endoscope-assisted microscopic resections are able to reach and remove more invasive tumor. In their series of 140 patients harboring 30 functional microadenomas, 39 functional macroadenomas, and 71 nonfunctional adenomas, endoscopy was able to identify additional tumor in 40% of patients following microscopic removal, resulting in additional tumor removal in 36% of cases. Notably, tumors measuring >2 cm in diameter underwent additional tumor removal in 54% of cases, including removal of residual invasive tumor from the medial cavernous sinus. They achieved an early remission rate of 70%, suggesting that superior visibility via the endoscopic approach results in improved surgical and endocrine outcomes.[42]

SURGICAL MANAGEMENT OF INVASIVE ADENOMAS

Numerous studies have demonstrated an association between cavernous sinus invasion and lesser extent of resection.[32,43–50] Importantly, the degree of cavernous sinus invasion varies drastically between patients and can be the determining factor in degree of tumor removal,[7,9,17,51,52] highlighting the importance of preoperative grading as a means of adjusting treatment goals, approaches, and optimizing patient counseling. Although the techniques and indications for invasive PA resection are expanding rapidly, most studies can be dichotomized by their use of predominately transsellar approaches that traverse the medial wall of the cavernous sinus, versus expanded transcavernous approaches that traverse the cavernous sinus anteriorly.

TRANSSELLAR APPROACHES VIA THE MEDIAL WALL OF THE CAVERNOUS SINUS

Whether done via a traditional microscopic or endonasal endoscopic technique, direct approaches to the sella make use of transsphenoidal access in conjunction with wide dural openings to allow for effective resection of intrasellar and extrasellar tumor extension. PAs invading the cavernous sinus can be sequentially removed, beginning with their intrasellar components and subsequently working laterally, where invasion through the medial wall can be visualized or palpated in an effort to pursue further extent of resection.[52–54] In this regard, many investigators have reported their experience in the removal of cavernous sinus disease via predominately transsellar approaches. The use of angled endoscopy to inspect and resect additional tumor from the medial cavernous sinus wall in this setting has been one of the major advantages of endoscopic endonasal approaches versus microscopic approaches.

In a large meta-analysis of 14 studies examining rates of biochemical remission among 972 patients treated surgically for somatotrophs, the authors found significantly lower rates of biochemical remission in invasive PAs versus noninvasive PAs (48% vs 76%).[55] Hofstetter and colleagues[53] report their experience in the management of 86 patients with functional PA who underwent endoscopic endonasal resection; 21% invaded the cavernous sinus. Of these invasive PAs, there was a 33.3% rate of gross total resection, a factor that was significantly related to rates of biochemical remission. Seven of 18 patients (39%) with invasive PAs reached biochemical remission, including 3 prolactinomas, 3 somatotrophs, and 1 corticotroph.[53] Ajlan and colleagues[52] studied a cohort of 176 total PAs treated predominately with the direct endoscopic approach and found a 23% rate of cavernous sinus invasion that diminished the odds of gross total resection from 86% for noninvasive tumors to 47% for those invading the cavernous sinus. Biochemical remission was achieved in just 15% of invasive PAs versus 63% of noninvasive PAs, although there was no difference in rates of complications, including CSF leak and cranial neuropathy.

Campbell and colleagues[56] examined their direct endoscopic experience in patients with acromegaly, noting that invasive tumors (Knosp grade ≥3) were less likely to experience biochemical remission. Patients with residual cavernous sinus disease underwent multimodality radiosurgery and medical treatment postoperatively. Similarly, Park and colleagues[57] found that somatotroph PAs encasing the cavernous ICA resulted in only 14.7% gross total remission, even when intracavernous tumor resection was attempted. On the other hand, Nishioka and colleagues[54] report excellent results with a predominately medial-to-lateral resection strategy, whereby the medial wall is opened aggressively and often laterally toward the anterior genu of the cavernous ICA, resulting in biochemical remission rates of 70% for the invasive somatotrophs in their series.

Giant, invasive PAs present a similar challenge for maximizing extent of resection and biochemical remission. De Paiva Neto and colleagues[47] found that invasive giant PAs (Knosp grade 3 or 4) were particularly difficult to cure with surgery, with only 9.6% of invasive cases undergoing gross total resection and a 0% biochemical remission rate for functional adenomas with surgery alone. Another series of giant, predominately nonfunctional PAs (defined here as ≥3 cm) found that, among 31 patients with Knosp grade 3 and 4 tumors, the mean volumetric extent of resection (EOR) was 78% and 69%, respectively.[58]

EXTENDED TRANSCAVERNOUS APPROACHES

Despite limited evidence that transcranial transcavernous approaches can be performed with low morbidity,[59–61] increasing endoscopic literature suggests the feasibility of expanded approaches to and through the cavernous sinus. Numerous investigators have explored the safety and utility of extended transcavernous approaches for invasive cavernous sinus disease.

In a cohort of Knosp grade 4 nonfunctional PA patients who underwent both transsellar, medial-to-lateral exposure and direct transcavernous exposure and resection, Toda and colleagues[62] were able to achieve near or gross total resection in 12 of 30 patients (40%), with an average volumetric EOR of 74%. They suggest a favorable safety profile with minimal morbidity, including CSF leak and meningitis occurring each in a single patient, and transient cranial neuropathy in 2 patients. Ceylan and colleagues[63] also used progressively more direct transcavernous approaches in their reported series of functional and nonfunctional PAs, achieving gross total resection rates of 65% for Knosp grade 3 and 4 PAs and biochemical remission in 75% of prolactinomas, 75% of corticotroph PAs, and 57% of somatotroph PAs. Bao and colleagues[64] report relatively high rates of resection with direct transcavernous approaches, including 92% for Knosp grade 3 PAs and 54% for Knosp grade 4 PAs, with an overall biochemical remission rate of 56% at 3 months, and a cranial neuropathy rate of 2.9% for first-time operations. Similarly, Zhao and colleagues[65] report rates of 91% and 48% for Knosp grade 3 and 4 PAs, respectively, using a combination of extended, direct transcavernous approaches. Although remission rates are likely to decrease with longer follow-up,[66] the low morbidity rates reported, including less than 1% ICA injury rate suggest that transcavernous approaches may provide higher rates of tumor and endocrinological control with acceptable morbidity.

In contrast to these investigators, some series reported lower rates of gross total resection and biochemical remission. Paluzzi and colleagues[8] reviewed their experience with the endoscopic management of 555 patients with PAs, including 165 (31.8%) who required direct transcavernous approaches for invasive disease; their overall gross total resection rate for macroadenomas with invasion (Knosp grades 2–4) was 35.4%, including biochemical remission rates of 47.4% for somatotroph PAs, 40% for corticotroph PAs, 17.6% for prolactinomas, and rates of cranial neuropathy and ICA injury less than 1%. Woodworth and colleagues[67] used a medial-to-lateral approach with entry into the cavernous sinus lateral to the ICA in 23 patients with Knosp grade 3 and 4 PAs, resulting in near or gross total resection for 3 patients (13%); 2 patients (8.7%) suffered transient cranial neuropathy.

In an effort to better systematize cavernous sinus invasion seen intraoperatively, Fernandez-Miranda and colleagues[51] developed an anatomic classification of cavernous sinus invasion specifically tailored to the endonasal endoscopic approach. Through use of cadaveric specimens, the authors established 4 intracavernous compartments based on the course of the cavernous carotid subsequently correlated with EOR: the superior compartment lies over the horizontal cavernous ICA and behind its genu, and is bounded by the interclinoidal ligament and oculomotor nerve; the posterior compartment is located between the vertical cavernous ICA and the petroclival dura that comprises the posterior cavernous sinus wall; the inferior compartment lies inferior to the horizontal and anterior genu segments of the cavernous ICA; the lateral compartment lies lateral to the anterior genu and horizontal cavernous ICA, bounded superiorly by the proximal dural ring and inferiorly by the maxillary strut. Twenty-nine patients showed tumor invasion into a single compartment, and the remaining 69 patients demonstrated invasion into multiple compartments; superior compartment invasion was most common in both cohorts. Notably, resection rates varied by compartment, with 38% of patients having residual tumor following transcavernous resection on postoperative MRI. The lateral compartment most commonly had residual disease (19 patients, 79%), followed by posterior (12 patients, 17%), superior (12 patients, 14%), and inferior (6 patients, 11%). Complications included transient abducens nerve paresis in 2 patients, postoperative hematoma in 3 patients resulting in visual disturbance, and 1 ICA injury. The authors concluded that transcavernous resection is feasible with low morbidity, and that such anatomic understanding facilitates greater EOR. In general, complication profiles in most large case series generally report rates less than 10%, including hypopituitarism less than 10%, CSF leak less than 7%, ophthalmoplegia less than 6%, and ICA injury less than 2%.[8,32,52,67,68]

Lastly, in select cases it may be possible to combine open and endoscopic techniques for the resection of giant adenomas, sometimes even simultaneously.[69–71] In select cases, combined approaches that incorporate open craniotomy can adequately debulk tumors to facilitate visual recovery, although EOR and endocrine recovery remain predictably poorer relative to smaller lesions treated with single approaches.[69–72]

RADIATION-BASED THERAPIES FOR INVASIVE PITUITARY ADENOMAS

In general, the goals of radiation for PAs are to achieve tumor control and induce biochemical remission. The focal nature of residual and/or inaccessible disease within the cavernous sinus has led multiple investigators to study the utility of Gamma Knife radiosurgery for functional and nonfunctional PAs. Although external beam radiotherapy delivered in daily fractions to a total dose of 40 to 45 Gy has shown long-term durability in most patients up to 30 years posttreatment,[73–76] the need for daily treatments, the risk of secondary malignancy, and the lengthy time until tumor control and biochemical remission makes it a less desirable option in many patients.[77] Furthermore, external beam radiation inherently cannot offer the precision and specificity that radiosurgery offers, and effects of radiation on the normal pituitary gland and optic apparatus may arise in a delayed fashion following treatment.

For these reasons, most providers currently use stereotactic radiosurgery (SRS) rather than external beam radiation, which offers more precise delivery of radiation with an ability to achieve higher dosages to the tumor in each fraction, while limiting dosing to the optic apparatus and pituitary gland. There is ample evidence that patients can achieve radiographic and endocrinologic control through use of SRS, although data for radiosurgically treated disease specifically within the cavernous sinus is somewhat more limited.

For invasive nonfunctional PAs, Sheehan and colleagues[78] achieved tumor control in 96% of patients with residual disease using a mean dose of 16 Gy and over a mean follow-up time of 31 months, with no new hypopituitarism. Liu and colleagues[79] reported tumor control rates of 67% with a mean prescribed dose of 12.4 Gy over a mean follow-up of 33 months.

Far more data exist for functional PAs treated with SRS for invasive disease. Among dopamine agonist-resistant or -intolerant patients with invasive prolactinomas, prolactin normalization can be achieved in 27.3% to 50% of patients following SRS, with tumor control achieved in 86% to 92% of patients.[80,81] For invasive somatotroph PAs, Ikeda and colleagues[82] reported a rate of 82% biochemical remission when treated using Gamma Knife radiosurgery. By comparison, Kim and colleagues[83] reported complete tumor control in all 30 patients they studied, including 83% whose tumor decreased in volume. Only 47% of patients achieved endocrine remission following Gamma Knife radiosurgery at a median of 35 months, although the percentage increased to 66% at 10-year follow-up among patients receiving medical therapy. Notably, postoperative hypopituitarism developed in 30% of patients, and radiation necrosis was seen in 13.8% of patients, highlighting that, although effective, SRS is not without risk for complications.[83] Similarly, Pai and colleagues[84] found that among 76 patients with acromegaly with just over half showing cavernous sinus invasion, biochemical remission was achieved in 43.4% following SRS. In another series of invasive somatotrophs, 20 Gy delivered to the tumor margin resulted in 40% biochemical remission at 2 years posttreatment, and growth arrest in all cases.[85]

Due possibly to the smaller size at presentation, there are few data on residual or inaccessible cavernous sinus corticotrophs that underwent SRS. In general, for corticotroph PAs treated using Gamma Knife radiosurgery, hormonal remission rates range from 17% to 87%, with rates of hypopituitarism reaching as high as 66%.[86,87] However, 1 study reporting outcomes following CyberKnife radiosurgery administered at a median prescribed dose of 25 Gy to 7 patients with corticotroph PAs that were recurrent or invasive into the cavernous sinus reported biochemical remission in 4 patients (57%) at a median of 12.5 months, with only 1 patient suffering hypopituitarism.[88] Tumor control was seen in all cases.

Among studies of multiple functional PA subtypes, Shin and colleagues[89] treated 3 nonfunctional and 13 functional PAs using 16 and 30 Gy, respectively; with a median follow-up of 3 years, no tumors progressed, there were no new cases of hypopituitarism or visual loss, and biochemical remission was seen in 66% of somatotroph PAs and 50% of corticotroph PAs. Petrovich and colleagues[77] described their experience in the management of 78 patients with recurrent or residual PAs, with 96% of patients harboring disease within the cavernous sinus. A median prescription dose of 15 Gy resulted in tumor shrinkage in all patients, and biochemical remission within 2 years was noted in 100% of somatotroph PAs, 83% of prolactinomas, and 50% of corticotroph PAs. Notably, 53% of patients with preoperative cranial nerve palsies showed improvement following SRS.[77] Kim and colleagues[90] reported tumor control rates of 96% and biochemical remission in 68% of patients with invasive PAs, over a mean follow-up of 33 months.

Interestingly, there are conflicting data regarding the relative radiosensitivity of different functional PA subtypes, with some publications reporting differences,[91–93] and others noting none.[94,95] In addition, the presence of invasion itself may be negatively correlated with treatment response,[84,91,92] and may predispose to postradiosurgery hypopituitarism,[81,96] possibly due to more difficult treatment volumes and dose delivery that invariably passes through the pituitary gland. For this reason, some investigators have attempted to surgically transpose the pituitary gland[97] in an effort to lessen the risk associated with SRS.

SUMMARY

Although the biological and pathologic mechanisms driving invasion remain incompletely understood, the clinical behavior of invasive PAs attests to the intrinsically more aggressive nature of these lesions. Even among invasive PAs that undergo gross total resection, their propensity to recur[98] suggests an inherent tendency for proliferation intermixed with their invasive behavior. Coupled with the challenging anatomy and surgical access of the cavernous sinus, the unique biology of invasive PAs demands multimodality approaches and novel treatment strategies. The promise of medical therapy, including dopamine agonists and somatostatin analogs, represents the final step toward curing invasive disease. Targeted treatment of prolactinomas, somatotrophs, and corticotrophs, which makes use of their unique biology and surface receptors,[99] has resulted in medically induced biochemical remission for all 3 classes of functional adenomas, often with minimal side effects.[100–107]

The increasingly diverse array of transcavernous techniques for resection highlights the ongoing growth of endoscopic skull base surgery, and advances in the application of SRS techniques and targeted therapy make previously unresectable disease now manageable, with favorable rates of tumor control and biochemical remission when multimodality approaches are taken.[8,32,47,52,63,67,68] Future studies that incorporate elements of all 3 modalities will undoubtedly offer patients with invasive PAs the best outcome.

REFERENCES

1. Hayashi Y, Sasagawa Y, Oishi M, et al. Directional regulation of extrasellar extension by sellar dura integrity and intrasphenoidal septation in pituitary adenomas. World Neurosurg 2018;122:e130–8.
2. Sarkar S, Chacko AG, Chacko G. Clinicopathological correlates of extrasellar growth patterns in pituitary adenomas. J Clin Neurosci 2015;22(7):1173–7.
3. Singh H, Essayed WI, Cohen-Gadol A, et al. Resection of pituitary tumors: endoscopic versus microscopic. J Neurooncol 2016;130(2):309–17.
4. Yoneoka Y, Watanabe N, Matsuzawa H, et al. Preoperative depiction of cavernous sinus invasion by pituitary macroadenoma using three-dimensional anisotropy contrast periodically rotated overlapping parallel lines with enhanced reconstruction imaging on a 3-tesla system. J Neurosurg 2008;108(1):37–41.
5. Ahmadi J, North CM, Segall HD, et al. Cavernous sinus invasion by pituitary adenomas. Am J Roentgenol 1986;146(2):257–62.
6. Fahlbusch R, Buchfelder M. Transsphenoidal surgery of parasellar pituitary adenomas. Acta Neurochir (Wien) 1988;92(1–4):93–9.
7. Knosp E, Steiner E, Kitz K, et al. Pituitary adenomas with invasion of the cavernous sinus space: a magnetic resonance imaging classification compared with surgical findings. Neurosurgery 1993;33(4):610–8.
8. Paluzzi A, Fernandez-Miranda JC, Tonya Stefko S, et al. Endoscopic endonasal approach for pituitary adenomas: a series of 555 patients. Pituitary 2014; 17(4):307–19.
9. Micko ASG, Wöhrer A, Wolfsberger S, et al. Invasion of the cavernous sinus space in pituitary adenomas: endoscopic verification and its correlation with an MRI-based classification. J Neurosurg 2015;122(4):803–11.
10. Campero A, Campero AA, Martins C, et al. Surgical anatomy of the dural walls of the cavernous sinus. J Clin Neurosci 2010;17(6):746–50.
11. Martins C, Yasuda A, Campero A, et al. Microsurgical anatomy of the oculomotor cistern. Neurosurgery 2006;58(SUPPL. 2). https://doi.org/10.1227/01.NEU.0000204673.55834.
12. Capo H, Kupersmith MJ, Berenstein A, et al. The clinical importance of the inferolateral trunk of the internal carotid artery. Neurosurgery 1991;28(5):733–8.
13. Oikawa S, Kyoshima K, Kobayashi S. Surgical anatomy of the juxta-dural ring area. J Neurosurg 1998;250–4. https://doi.org/10.3171/jns.1998.89.2.0250.
14. Campero A, Martins C, Yasuda A, et al. Microsurgical anatomy of the diaphragma sellae and its role in directing the pattern of growth of pituitary adenomas. Neurosurgery 2008;62(3):717–22.
15. Yokoyama S, Hirano H, Moroki K, et al. Are nonfunctioning pituitary adenomas extending into the cavernous sinus aggressive and/or invasive? Neurosurgery 2001;49(4):857–62 [discussion: 862–3]. Available at: http://www.ncbi.nlm.nih.gov/pubmed/11564246. Accessed July 25, 2015.
16. Sasagawa Y, Tachibana O, Doai M, et al. Internal carotid arterial shift after transsphenoidal surgery in pituitary adenomas with cavernous sinus invasion. Pituitary 2013;16(4):465–70.
17. Chotai S, Liu Y, Qi S. Review of surgical anatomy of the tumors involving cavernous sinus. Asian J Neurosurg 2018;13(1):1.
18. Vieira JO, Cukiert A, Liberman B. Evaluation of magnetic resonance imaging criteria for cavernous sinus invasion in patients with pituitary adenomas: logistic regression analysis and correlation with surgical findings. Surg Neurol 2006; 65(2):130–5.
19. Connor SEJ, Wilson F, Hogarth K. Magnetic resonance imaging criteria to predict complete excision of parasellar pituitary macroadenoma on postoperative imaging. J Neurol Surg B Skull Base 2014; 75(1):41–6.
20. Trevisi G, Vigo V, Morena MG, et al. Comparison of endoscopic versus microsurgical resection of pituitary adenomas with parasellar extension and evaluation of the predictive value of a simple 4-quadrant radiologic classification. World Neurosurg 2018;121:e769–74.
21. Mohr G, Hardy J, Comtois R, et al. Surgical management of giant pituitary adenomas. Can J Neurol Sci 1990;17(1):62–6.

22. Mooney MA, Hardesty DA, Sheehy JP, et al. Rater reliability of the hardy classification for pituitary adenomas in the magnetic resonance imaging era. J Neurol Surg B Skull Base 2017;78(5): 413–8.

23. Hardy J, Vezina JL. Transsphenoidal neurosurgery of intracranial neoplasm. Adv Neurol 1976;15: 261–73. Available at: http://www.ncbi.nlm.nih.gov/pubmed/945663.

24. Mooney MA, Hardesty DA, Sheehy JP, et al. Inter-rater and intrarater reliability of the Knosp scale for pituitary adenoma grading. J Neurosurg 2017; 126(5):1714–9.

25. Ammirati M, Wei L, Ciric I. Short-term outcome of endoscopic versus microscopic pituitary adenoma surgery: a systematic review and meta-analysis. J Neurol Neurosurg Psychiatry 2013;84(8):843–9.

26. Dallapiazza R, Bond AE, Grober Y, et al. Retrospective analysis of a concurrent series of microscopic versus endoscopic transsphenoidal surgeries for Knosp Grades 0–2 nonfunctioning pituitary macroadenomas at a single institution. J Neurosurg 2014;121(3):511–7.

27. Pal'a A, Knoll A, Brand C, et al. The value of intraoperative magnetic resonance imaging in endoscopic and microsurgical transsphenoidal pituitary adenoma resection. World Neurosurg 2017;102:144–50.

28. Zaidi HA, Cote DJ, Dunn IF, et al. Predictors of aggressive clinical phenotype among immunohistochemically confirmed atypical adenomas. J Clin Neurosci 2016. https://doi.org/10.1016/j.jocn.2016.09.014.

29. Esquenazi Y, Essayed WI, Singh H, et al. Endoscopic endonasal versus microscopic transsphenoidal surgery for recurrent and/or residual pituitary adenomas. World Neurosurg 2017;101: 186–95.

30. Messerer M, De battista JC, Raverot G, et al. Evidence of improved surgical outcome following endoscopy for nonfunctioning pituitary adenoma removal. Neurosurg Focus 2011;E11. https://doi.org/10.3171/2011.1.FOCUS10308.

31. Wang A, Shah A, Sidani C, et al. Volumetry in the assessment of pituitary adenoma resection: endoscopy versus microscopy. J Neurol Surg B Skull Base 2018;79(06):538–44.

32. Dhandapani S, Singh H, Negm HM, et al. Cavernous sinus invasion in pituitary adenomas: systematic review and pooled data meta-analysis of radiologic criteria and comparison of endoscopic and microscopic surgery. World Neurosurg 2016;96:36–46.

33. Li A, Liu W, Cao P, et al. Endoscopic versus microscopic transsphenoidal surgery in the treatment of pituitary adenoma: a systematic review and meta-analysis. World Neurosurg 2017;101:236–46.

34. Gao Y, Zhong C, Wang Y, et al. Endoscopic versus microscopic transsphenoidal pituitary adenoma surgery: a meta-analysis. World J Surg Oncol 2014;12(1). https://doi.org/10.1186/1477-7819-12-94.

35. Yu SY, Du Q, Yao SY, et al. Outcomes of endoscopic and microscopic transsphenoidal surgery on non-functioning pituitary adenomas: a systematic review and meta-analysis. J Cell Mol Med 2018;22(3):2023–7.

36. Sylvester PT, Evans JA, Zipfel GJ, et al. Combined high-field intraoperative magnetic resonance imaging and endoscopy increase extent of resection and progression-free survival for pituitary adenomas. Pituitary 2015;18(1):72–85.

37. Almutairi RD, Muskens IS, Cote DJ, et al. Gross total resection of pituitary adenomas after endoscopic vs. microscopic transsphenoidal surgery: a meta-analysis. Acta Neurochir (Wien) 2018; 160(5):1005–21.

38. Negm HM, Al-Mahfoudh R, Pai M, et al. Reoperative endoscopic endonasal surgery for residual or recurrent pituitary adenomas. J Neurosurg 2016; 1–12. https://doi.org/10.3171/2016.8.JNS152709.

39. Broersen LHA, Biermasz NR, van Furth WR, et al. Endoscopic vs. microscopic transsphenoidal surgery for Cushing's disease: a systematic review and meta-analysis. Pituitary 2018;21(5):524–34.

40. D'Haens J, Van Rompaey K, Stadnik T, et al. Fully endoscopic transsphenoidal surgery for functioning pituitary adenomas. A retrospective comparison with traditional transsphenoidal microsurgery in the same institution. Surg Neurol 2009;72(4):336–40.

41. Wagenmakers MAEM, Boogaarts HD, Roerink SHPP, et al. Endoscopic transsphenoidal pituitary surgery: a good and safe primary treatment option for Cushing's disease, even in case of macroadenomas or invasive adenomas. Eur J Endocrinol 2013;169(3): 329–37.

42. McLaughlin N, Eisenberg AA, Cohan P, et al. Value of endoscopy for maximizing tumor removal in endonasal transsphenoidal pituitary adenoma surgery. J Neurosurg 2013;118(3):613–20.

43. Karamouzis I, Caputo M, Mele C, et al. Transsphenoidal surgery for pituitary adenomas: early results from a single center. Hormones 2018. https://doi.org/10.1007/s42000-018-0082-9.

44. Meij BP, Lopes M-BS, Ellegala DB, et al. The long-term significance of microscopic dural invasion in 354 patients with pituitary adenomas treated with transsphenoidal surgery. J Neurosurg 2002;96(2): 195–208.

45. Serra C, Staartjes VE, Maldaner N, et al. Predicting extent of resection in transsphenoidal surgery for pituitary adenoma. Acta Neurochir (Wien) 2018; 160(11):2255–62.

46. Messerer M, Daniel RT, Cossu G. No doubt: the invasion of the cavernous sinus is the limiting factor for complete resection in pituitary adenomas. Acta Neurochir (Wien) 2019. https://doi.org/10.1007/s00701-018-03784-2.

47. De Paiva Neto MA, Vandergrift A, Fatemi N, et al. Endonasal transsphenoidal surgery and multimodality treatment for giant pituitary adenomas. Clin Endocrinol (Oxf) 2010;72(4):512–9.

48. Elshazly K, Kshettry VR, Farrell CJ, et al. Clinical outcomes after endoscopic endonasal resection of giant pituitary adenomas. World Neurosurg 2018;114:e447–56.

49. Sanmillán JL, Torres-Diaz A, Sanchez-Fernández JJ, et al. Radiologic predictors for extent of resection in pituitary adenoma surgery. A single-center study. World Neurosurg 2017;108: 436–46.

50. Hwang J, Seol HJ, Nam D-H, et al. Therapeutic strategy for cavernous sinus-invading non-functioning pituitary adenomas based on the modified Knosp grading system. Brain Tumor Res Treat 2016;4(2):63.

51. Fernandez-Miranda JC, Zwagerman NT, Abhinav K, et al. Cavernous sinus compartments from the endoscopic endonasal approach: anatomical considerations and surgical relevance to adenoma surgery. J Neurosurg 2017;1–12. https://doi.org/10.3171/2017.2.JNS162214.

52. Ajlan A, Achrol A, Albakr A, et al. Cavernous sinus involvement by pituitary adenomas: clinical implications and outcomes of endoscopic endonasal resection. J Neurol Surg B Skull Base 2017; 38(03):273 82.

53. Hofstetter CP, Shin BJ, Mubita L, et al. Endoscopic endonasal transsphenoidal surgery for functional pituitary adenomas. Neurosurg Focus 2011;30(4): E10.

54. Nishioka H, Fukuhara N, Horiguchi K, et al. Aggressive transsphenoidal resection of tumors invading the cavernous sinus in patients with acromegaly: predictive factors, strategies, and outcomes. J Neurosurg 2014;121(3):505–10.

55. Briceno V, Zaidi HA, Doucette JA, et al. Efficacy of transsphenoidal surgery in achieving biochemical cure of growth hormone-secreting pituitary adenomas among patients with cavernous sinus invasion: a systematic review and meta-analysis. Neurol Res 2017;39(5):387–98.

56. Campbell PG, Kenning E, Andrews DW, et al. Outcomes after a purely endoscopic transsphenoidal resection of growth hormone-secreting pituitary adenomas. Neurosurg Focus 2010;29(4):E5.

57. Park HH, Kim EH, Ku CR, et al. Outcomes of aggressive surgical resection in growth hormone-secreting pituitary adenomas with cavernous sinus invasion. World Neurosurg 2018;117:e280–9.

58. Juraschka K, Khan OH, Godoy BL, et al. Endoscopic endonasal transsphenoidal approach to large and giant pituitary adenomas: institutional experience and predictors of extent of resection. J Neurosurg 2014;121(1):75–83.

59. Spallone A, Vidal R, Gonzales J. Transcranial approach to pituitary adenomas invading the cavernous sinus: a modification of the classical technique to be used in a low-technology environment. Surg Neurol Int 2010;1(1):25.

60. Tamiya T, Ono Y, Date I, et al. [Extradural temporopolar approach for giant pituitary adenomas invading the cavernous sinus and parasellar regions]. No Shinkei Geka 1998;26(9):803–11. Available at: http://www.ncbi.nlm.nih.gov/pubmed/9757457.

61. Hakuba A, Tanaka K, Suzuki T, et al. A combined orbitozygomatic infratemporal epidural and subdural approach for lesions involving the entire cavernous sinus. J Neurosurg 1989;71(5 Pt 1): 699–704.

62. Toda M, Kosugi K, Ozawa H, et al. Surgical treatment of cavernous sinus lesion in patients with nonfunctioning pituitary adenomas via the endoscopic endonasal approach. J Neurol Surg B Skull Base 2018;79(Suppl 4):S311–5.

63. Ceylan S, Koc K, Anik I. Endoscopic endonasal transsphenoidal approach for pituitary adenomas invading the cavernous sinus. J Neurosurg 2010; 99–107. https://doi.org/10.3171/2009.4.JNS09182.

64. Bao X, Deng K, Liu X, et al. Extended transsphenoidal approach for pituitary adenomas invading the cavernous sinus using multiple complementary techniques. Pituitary 2016;19(1):1–10.

65. Zhao B, Wei Y-K, Li G-L, et al. Extended transsphenoidal approach for pituitary adenomas invading the anterior cranial base, cavernous sinus, and clivus: a single-center experience with 126 consecutive cases. J Neurosurg 2010;108–17. https://doi.org/10.3171/2009.3.JNS0929.

66. Oldfield EH. Editorial: management of invasion by pituitary adenomas. J Neurosurg 2014;121(3): 501–4.

67. Woodworth GF, Patel KS, Shin B, et al. Surgical outcomes using a medial-to-lateral endonasal endoscopic approach to pituitary adenomas invading the cavernous sinus. J Neurosurg 2014;120(5): 1086–94.

68. Koutourousiou M, Vaz Guimaraes Filho F, Fernandez-Miranda JC, et al. Endoscopic endonasal surgery for tumors of the cavernous sinus: a series of 234 patients. World Neurosurg 2017;103: 713–32.

69. Kuga D, Toda M, Ozawa H, et al. Endoscopic endonasal approach combined with a simultaneous transcranial approach for giant pituitary tumors. World Neurosurg 2019;121:173–9.

70. Kroppenstedt SN, Blumenthal DT, Niepage S, et al. Combined transsphenoidal and pterional craniotomy approach to giant pituitary tumors. Surg Neurol 2002;57(6):380–90.

71. Leung GKK, Yuen MMA, Chow WS, et al. An endoscopic modification of the simultaneous "above and below" approach to large pituitary adenomas. Pituitary 2012;15(2):237–41.

72. Leung GKK, Law HY, Hung KN, et al. Combined simultaneous transcranial and transsphenoidal resection of large-to-giant pituitary adenomas. Acta Neurochir (Wien) 2011;153(7):1401–8.

73. Grigsby PW, Simpson JR, Fineberg B. Late regrowth of pituitary adenomas after irradiation and/or surgery. Hazard function analysis. Cancer 1989;63(7):1308–12.

74. Breen P, Flickinger JC, Kondziolka D, et al. Radiotherapy for nonfunctional pituitary adenoma: analysis of long-term tumor control. J Neurosurg 1998;89(6):933–8.

75. Hughes MN, Llamas KJ, Yelland ME, et al. Pituitary adenomas: long-term results for radiotherapy alone and post-operative radiotherapy. Int J Radiat Oncol Biol Phys 1993;27(5):1035–43.

76. Haghighi N, Seely A, Paul E, et al. Hypofractionated stereotactic radiotherapy for benign intracranial tumours of the cavernous sinus. J Clin Neurosci 2015;22(9):1450–5.

77. Petrovich Z, Yu C, Giannotta SL, et al. Gamma knife radiosurgery for pituitary adenoma: early results. Neurosurgery 2003;53(1):51–61.

78. Sheehan JP, Kondziolka D, Flickinger J, et al. Radiosurgery for residual or recurrent nonfunctioning pituitary adenoma. J Neurosurg 2002;97(5 Suppl):408–14.

79. Liu AL, Wang C, Sun S, et al. Gamma knife radiosurgery for tumors involving the cavernous sinus. Stereotact Funct Neurosurg 2005;83(1):45–51.

80. Liu X, Kano H, Kondziolka D, et al. Gamma knife stereotactic radiosurgery for drug resistant or intolerant invasive prolactinomas. Pituitary 2013;16(1):68–75.

81. Cohen-Inbar O, Xu Z, Schlesinger D, et al. Gamma Knife radiosurgery for medically and surgically refractory prolactinomas: long-term results. Pituitary 2015;18(6):820–30.

82. Ikeda H, Jokura H, Yoshimoto T. Transsphenoidal surgery and adjuvant gamma knife treatment for growth hormone-secreting pituitary adenoma. J Neurosurg 2001;95(2):285–91.

83. Kim EH, Oh MC, Chang JH, et al. Postoperative gamma knife radiosurgery for cavernous sinus-invading growth hormone-secreting pituitary adenomas. World Neurosurg 2018;110:e534–45.

84. Pai F-Y, Chen C-J, Wang W-H, et al. Low-dose gamma knife radiosurgery for acromegaly. Neurosurgery 2018. https://doi.org/10.1093/neuros/nyy410.

85. Fukuoka S, Ito T, Takanashi M, et al. Gamma knife radiosurgery for growth hormone-secreting pituitary adenomas invading the cavernous sinus. Stereotact Funct Neurosurg 2001;76:213–7.

86. Höybye C, Grenbäck E, Rähn T, et al. Adrenocorticotropic hormone-producing pituitary tumors: 12- to 22-year follow-up after treatment with stereotactic radiosurgery. Neurosurgery 2001;49(2):284–92.

87. Minniti G, Clarke E, Scaringi C, et al. Stereotactic radiotherapy and radiosurgery for non-functioning and secreting pituitary adenomas. Rep Pract Oncol Radiother 2016;21(4):370–8.

88. Moore JM, Sala E, Amorin A, et al. CyberKnife radiosurgery in the multimodal management of patients with Cushing disease. World Neurosurg 2018;112:e425–30.

89. Shin M, Kurita H, Sasaki T, et al. Stereotactic radiosurgery for pituitary adenoma invading the cavernous sinus. J Neurosurg 2000;93(Suppl 3):2–5.

90. Kim M, Paeng S, Pyo S, et al. Gamma Knife surgery for invasive pituitary macroadenoma. J Neurosurg 2006;26–30. https://doi.org/10.3171/sup.2006.105.7.26.

91. Pamir MN, Kiliç T, Belirgen M, et al. Pituitary adenomas treated with gamma knife radiosurgery: volumetric analysis of 100 cases with minimum 3 year follow-up. Neurosurgery 2007;61(2):270–80.

92. Trifiletti DM, Xu Z, Dutta SW, et al. Endocrine remission after pituitary stereotactic radiosurgery: differences in rates of response for matched cohorts of Cushing disease and acromegaly patients. Int J Radiat Oncol Biol Phys 2018;101(3):610–7.

93. Pollock BE, Brown PD, Nippoldt TB, et al. Pituitary tumor type affects the chance of biochemical remission after radiosurgery of hormone-secreting pituitary adenomas. Neurosurgery 2008;62(6):1271–8.

94. Pollock BE, Nippoldt TB, Stafford SL, et al. Results of stereotactic radiosurgery in patients with hormone-producing pituitary adenomas: factors associated with endocrine normalization. J Neurosurg 2002;525–30. https://doi.org/10.3171/jns.2002.97.3.0525.

95. Lee CC, Vance ML, Lopes MB, et al. Stereotactic radiosurgery for acromegaly: outcomes by adenoma subtype. Pituitary 2015;18(3):326–34.

96. Cohen-Inbar O, Ramesh A, Xu Z, et al. Gamma knife radiosurgery in patients with persistent acromegaly or Cushing's disease: long-term risk of hypopituitarism. Clin Endocrinol (Oxf) 2016;84(4):524–31.

97. Liu JK, Couldwell WT. Contemporary management of prolactinomas. Neurosurg Focus 2004;16(4):E2. Available at: http://www.ncbi.nlm.nih.gov/pubmed/15191331.

98. Lv L, Zhang B, Wang M, et al. Invasive pituitary adenomas with gross total resection: The wait-and-see policy during postoperative management. J Clin Neurosci 2018;58:49–55.

99. Mooney MA, Simon ED, Little AS. Advancing treatment of pituitary adenomas through targeted molecular therapies: the acromegaly and Cushing disease paradigms. Front Surg 2016;3. https://doi.org/10.3389/fsurg.2016.00045.

100. Dos Santos Nunes V, El Dib R, Boguszewski CL, et al. Cabergoline versus bromocriptine in the treatment of hyperprolactinemia: a systematic review of randomized controlled trials and meta-analysis. Pituitary 2011;14(3):259–65.

101. Wang AT, Mullan RJ, Lane MA, et al. Treatment of hyperprolactinemia: a systematic review and meta-analysis. Syst Rev 2006;1(1). https://doi.org/10.1186/2046-4053-1-33.

102. Wu ZB, Yu CJ, Su ZP, et al. Bromocriptine treatment of invasive giant prolactinomas involving the cavernous sinus: results of a long-term follow up. J Neurosurg 2006;54–61. https://doi.org/10.3171/jns.2006.104.1.54.

103. Yamamoto R, Robert Shima K, Igawa H, et al. Impact of preoperative pasireotide therapy on invasive octreotide-resistant acromegaly. Endocr J 2018;65(10):1061–7.

104. Manjila S, Wu OC, Khan FR, et al. Pharmacological management of acromegaly: a current perspective. Neurosurg Focus 2010;29(4):E14.

105. Rutkowski MJ, Breshears JD, Kunwar S, et al. Approach to the postoperative patient with Cushing's disease. Pituitary 2015;18(2). https://doi.org/10.1007/s11102-015-0644-7.

106. Oh MC, Aghi MK. Dopamine agonist-resistant prolactinomas. J Neurosurg 2011;114(5):1369–79.

107. Aghi MK. Management of recurrent and refractory Cushing disease. Nat Clin Pract Endocrinol Metab 2008;4(10):560–8.

Pituitary Apoplexy

Garni Barkhoudarian, MD[a,b,*], Daniel F. Kelly, MD[a,b]

KEYWORDS

• Pituitary apoplexy • Pituitary adenomas • Hypopituitarism • Headache • Diplopia • Vision loss

KEY POINTS

- Pituitary apoplexy is a clinical diagnosis requiring both acute onset of symptoms including vision loss, hypopituitarism, and/or severe headaches, as well as a hemorrhagic or infarcted pituitary lesion.
- Urgent management of hypopituitarism with hormone replacement is critical.
- The urgency of resection of the hemorrhagic pituitary adenomas or cyst depends on the severity and duration of symptoms.

INTRODUCTION - DEFINITION AND CLINICAL PRESENTATION

Pituitary apoplexy is a serious yet uncommon condition affecting patients with pituitary lesions. Most often, patients present with a hemorrhagic pituitary adenomas, although pituitary tumor infarctions can also present as apoplexy. Less often, intrasellar cysts, primarily Rathke cleft cysts, can rupture, causing pituitary inflammation and apoplexy symptoms.

Pituitary apoplexy affects 0.2% to 0.6% of the general population and can vary, affecting between 2% and 12% of patients with pituitary adenomas.[1–4] Presenting symptoms can be grouped into 3 major categories: vision, endocrine, and headaches.[5] The incidence of symptom presentation is list in **Table 1** (based on a large literature review by Breit and colleagues[4]).

MANAGEMENT

The approach for the management of pituitary apoplexy has been mired by dogma and pedigree. Treatment strategies have spanned from conservative management (cool off and observe) to emergent surgical resection. The philosophy of urgent surgical resection is extrapolated from intracranial hematoma surgery (acute subdural or epidural hematoma), where early relief of mass effect has demonstrated superior clinical outcomes in the setting of brain compression.

Conversely, the strategy of delayed surgical resection or observation has been predicated upon the fact that often these hemorrhagic pituitary adenomas are completely infarcted, and hence the hematoma will resorb and the underlying etiology be obliterated. This is similar to the approach for smaller intraparenchymal hematomas, which are often observed with good outcomes (ICH score 0 or 1).[6]

Both strategies have been employed with varying levels of success. Geographically, practice implementation has been variable, with conservative approaches more common in European countries and early surgical strategies more common in the United States. Given the obvious challenges of a prospective, blinded, and randomized controlled study to answer this question, the data to support any recommendations are class III, based on cohort analysis and expert consensus. Currently, there is an effort to prospectively analyze these treatment strategies via a large, multi-institution data registry (PASTOR – Pituitary Apoplexy Surgical Timing & Outcomes Registry).

Disclosure Statement: None.
[a] John Wayne Cancer Institute, Santa Monica, CA, USA; [b] Pacific Neuroscience Institute, 2125 Arizona Avenue, Santa Monica, CA 90404, USA
* Corresponding author. Pacific Neuroscience Institute, 2125 Arizona Avenue, Santa Monica, CA 90404.
E-mail address: BarkhoudarianG@jwci.org

Neurosurg Clin N Am 30 (2019) 457–463
https://doi.org/10.1016/j.nec.2019.06.001

Table 1
Incidence of presenting symptoms with pituitary apoplexy

Symptom	Incidence (%)
Headaches	73
Visual acuity loss	68
Hypopituitarism	64
Visual field loss	49
Nausea	49
Oculoparesis (diplopia)	48
Altered level of consciousness/ coma	17

Data from Briet C, Salevave S, Bonneville J, et al. Pituitary apoplexy. Endocr Rev. 2015 Dec;36(6):622-45.

This article discusses the authors' institutional approach to pituitary apoplexy patients, which is well accepted in many large pituitary centers of excellence and is supported by the existing literature.[7] Ultimately, the decision to proceed with surgery as well as the pace to do so is a product of the severity of the patient's symptoms and the duration of symptom presentation. This can be divided into 2 categories: acute and subacute (delayed) presentation.

Acute Presentation

The classic triad of symptoms in a patient presenting with pituitary apoplexy is severe, sudden-onset headache ("Worst headache of my life!"), acute hypopituitarism (Addisonian crisis, hyponatremia), and vision loss or visual disturbance (decreased visual acuity, decreased visual fields, and/or diplopia) – **Table 2**. Acute symptoms are defined as occurring within 24 to 72 hours. When these acute symptoms are identified, a pituitary protocol MRI should be obtained. If acute hemorrhage is noted on imaging (**Fig. 1**), then a diagnosis of pituitary apoplexy can be concluded. A hemorrhagic

Table 2
Classic triad of pituitary apoplexy symptoms

Sudden-onset headache	"Worst headache of my life!"
Addisonian crisis/shock	Severe fatigue, nausea, abdominal pain, hypotension, and altered mental status
Sudden-onset vision loss/disturbance	Decreased visual acuity, decreased visual fields, diplopia

pituitary tumor in the absence of these symptoms (currently and in the past) should not be categorized as pituitary apoplexy. Pituitary apoplexy is primarily a clinical diagnosis and relies on imaging solely as an adjunct to support this diagnosis.

For any patient with suspected pituitary apoplexy, in addition to a pituitary protocol MRI, a thorough neurologic examination should be performed, as well as a comprehensive laboratory analysis to include all pituitary hormones (**Table 3**). The neurologic examination should include a thorough cranial nerve evaluation, focusing on cranial nerves II to VI. Fundoscopic evaluation should be performed in the acute setting, focusing on identifying either papilledema or optic atrophy. Visual field assessment and optical coherence tomography (OCT) should be performed if available in the inpatient setting.[8] However, one should not delay intervention to acquire these studies, especially if there is clinical evidence of vision loss.

Preoperative management of these patients should include medical resuscitation when necessary and hormone replacement in the setting of hypopituitarism. The hypothalamic/pituitary/adrenal axis (HPA) should be addressed emergently. Hydrocortisone is the steroid of choice, given its physiologic similarity to cortisol, and stress doses are given up front, with supraphysiologic maintenance doses perioperatively. After surgery and after symptom recovery, this can be tapered to physiologic doses (**Table 4**).

In patients with pan-hypopituitarism, it is imperative to replace cortisol prior to replacing thyroid hormone. If thyroid hormone is replaced too early, the patient's metabolic rate may be increased without the HPA capacity to sustain it. This can tip the patient into Addisonian shock.[9] Hence, thyroid replacement is delayed by 24 hours after cortisol replacement is initiated.

Often, patients with pituitary apoplexy present with hyponatremia.[10] The most common diagnosis is the syndrome of inappropriate antidiuretic hormone (SIADH). The underlying etiology for SIADH in this patient population is acute hypocortisolism and hypothyroidism. Hence, correcting these hormone deficiencies will help correct the hyponatremia. Nevertheless, correcting the hyponatremia is pertinent, especially with low serum sodium concentrations (<125 mEq/L) and/or when the patient is symptomatic (nausea, vomiting, altered mental status). The hyponatremia should be correctly slowly (0.5 mEq/h or 12 mEq/d) to avoid intracranial osmolar shifts resulting in either central pontine myelinolysis (CPM) or extrapontine myelinolysis (EPM), both of which can cause severe and often permanent neurologic deficits.[11,12]

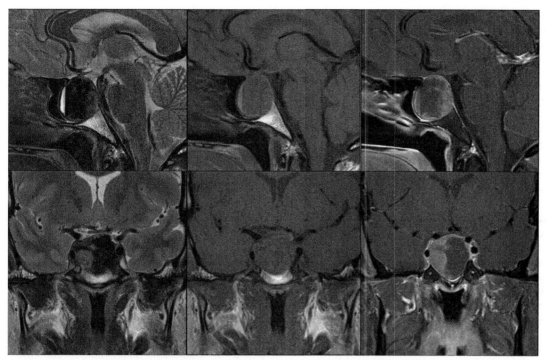

Fig. 1. Sagittal and coronal pituitary protocol MRI in a patient with acute pituitary hemorrhage (presented with clinical signs/symptoms of apoplexy). T1, T2, and postgadolineum T1 images are displayed.

MANAGEMENT OF ACUTE APOPLEXY

Once the patient is stabilized medically and is deemed to be an appropriate surgical candidate (eg, no major cardiac or pulmonary comorbidity), urgent or emergent surgical resection of the hemorrhagic pituitary tumor should be performed. The timing of surgery (whether to perform immediately or to wait until the morning) depends on the presence of vision loss and neurologic extremis. Any patient with acute-onset vision loss (whether decreased visual acuity or visual fields) who presents to the hospital within 24 to 72 hours of symptom onset should be treated emergently. Patients with new-onset diplopia in the absence of vision loss should be considered for emergent surgery, although overall recovery is good with surgical resection at any early time-point.[13] Patients with

Table 3
Pituitary hormone panel

Pituitary Hormone	Effector Hormone
Adrenocorticotropic hormone (ACTH)	Cortisol (fasting morning serum cortisol)
Thyroid-stimulating hormone (TSH)	Thyroxine (free T4 and free T3)
Growth hormone (GH)	Insulin-like growth factor (iGF-1)
Follicle stimulating hormone (FSH)	Progesterone (females)
Luteinizing hormone (LH)	Estrogen (females), testosterone (males)
Prolactin	No effector hormone
Antidiuretic hormone (ADH) (not measured clinically)	Assess serum sodium and serum/urine osmolarity.

Table 4
Hydrocortisone replacement strategy based on phase of care

Phase of Care	Hydrocortisone Dosing
Emergency room/ preoperative	50 mg every 8 hours
Perioperative (POD 1 and/or 2)	40 mg every morning/ 20 mg every evening
Maintenance (POD 3 and beyond)	20 mg every morning/ 10 mg every evening Or 10 mg every morning/5 mg daily at noon/5 mg every evening

only headaches or hypopituitarism can be treated symptomatically until surgery can be scheduled with a dedicated pituitary surgery team. If the prolactin level is suggestive of prolactinoma (>200 µg/L) and the patient has no acute and/or severe vision loss, then medical therapy with cabergoline maybe indicated as first-line therapy.[14]

Vision recovery (improvement of visual acuity or visual fields) and oculoparesis recovery are robust following pituitary apoplexy surgery. Between 74% and 94% of visual field/acuity deficits improve following surgery, although complete normal vision is achieved at a lower rate.[3,15,16] Oculoparesis recovery is more varied, ranging between 68% and 100%. Hormone recovery following surgery for pituitary apoplexy, however, is not as robust as with vision improvement. This is primarily because most patients present with some degree of pituitary dysfunction (64%–88%).[4,16,17] The chance of pituitary function improvement ranges from 12% to 23% depending on time of assessment.[15,16,18] Interestingly, Marcet and colleagues[17] report only a 14.7% rate of hormone replacement therapy following pituitary apoplexy surgery, suggesting dysfunction in the less vital axes (gonadotrophs or somatotrophs).

Goals of surgery are listed in **Table 5**. The surgical technique (whether microscopic or endoscopic) has not been demonstrated to have an impact on overall outcomes after pituitary apoplexy.[15,19] Ideally, patients should be treated by a high-volume pituitary surgery team.[7] However, in acute situations, surgical decompression and evacuation of hematoma should be attempted, with a definitive tumor resection deferred if necessary, at a pituitary center of excellence.

Postoperative management should include monitoring serum sodium levels to assess for SIADH and diabetes insipidus (DI). Hydrocortisone and levothyroxine should be maintained and tapered to physiologic doses prior to discharge. Assessment for durable skull base repair should be performed prior to discharge (tip test, postoperative computed tomography [CT] or MRI).

Subacute Presentation

Because of various circumstances, patients may not present in the acute phase (within 24–72 hours of symptom onset). This can be because of a lack of recognition of symptoms, lack of resources or access to tertiary care centers, mild symptoms, or short duration of symptoms. A typical patient may have a sudden onset headache 1 week prior to evaluation, treated with anti-inflammatory medications with partial resolution. Vision loss may not be recognized by patient, but can be detect on neurologic examination. Laboratory evaluation may demonstrate partial hypopituitarism. Imaging may demonstrate acute hemorrhage or infarction, but may also demonstrate subacute signs such as fluid-fluid levels or high T2-signal (**Fig. 2**).[20]

MANAGEMENT OF SUBACUTE APOPLEXY

Clearly the primary goal remains patient resuscitation, and hydrocortisone replacement is paramount for those with HPA axis deficiency. However, once the patient has been stabilized, the decision for management can be variable. Given the pathophysiology of apoplexy can result in tumor infarction, a large percentage of patients may not require surgical resection, and a conservative approach may be prudent.[21–23] However, there is a significant minority of patients who not only harbor viable tumor, but are at risk of further apoplexy.[24] Hence, a comprehensive analysis of the patient's condition should be considered, and the decision for surgery or conservative management should be made in concert with the patient's opinions and goals.

Patients that may be at higher risk for worse outcome include those with large hemorrhage, patients on long-term anticoagulation or with coagulopathy, patients with severe vision loss (dense bitemporal hemianopsia), and patients with invasive tumors. Interestingly, pituitary dysfunction, headaches, and oculomotor dysfunction tend to resolve over time with conservative management.[25] If surgery is

Table 5
Goals of surgery for acute and subacute onset pituitary apoplexy

	Acute Presentation	Sub-acute Presentation
1	Decompress optic apparatus, pituitary gland, and cavernous sinus	Maximal safe tumor resection
2	Evacuate hematoma	Decompression of optic apparatus, pituitary gland, and cavernous sinus
3	Resect tumor or cyst	Repair skull-base defect
4	Repair skull base defect	

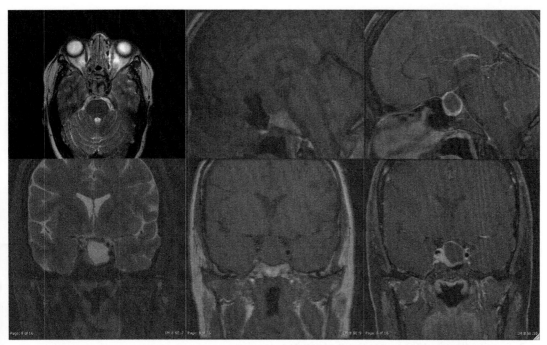

Fig. 2. Sagittal and coronal pituitary protocol MRI in a patient with subacute pituitary hemorrhage.

recommended in this setting, the goals of surgery are somewhat different than in the acute setting (see **Table 5**). Given the decreased urgency for these patients, surgical resection should be performed by a high-volume pituitary surgical team, ideally at a pituitary center of excellence with a multidisciplinary approach for perioperative care. If a conservative approach is elected, close monitoring is recommended, including repeat pituitary MRI, visual field test, and endocrine function tests.

SURGERY VERSUS CONSERVATIVE MANAGEMENT

There several studies that directly compare conservative and surgical management of pituitary apoplexy.[23,25–30] Given that none are randomized, controlled studies, the 2 populations cannot be compared appropriately. When the pituitary apoplexy score (PAS)[31] was applied (in only 1 of these studies - Bujawa Bujawansa and colleagues[32]), there was a clear discrimination between the conservative and surgical cohorts (1.8 v 3.8). Nevertheless, visual outcomes are equivocal between both groups. Interestingly, Tu and colleagues noted an improved in ocular palsy compared with conservative management, but did not note a difference in visual acuity or visual field analysis. Endocrine recovery was also equivocal, although Liu and colleagues[18] note a

slightly lower dependence on hormone replacement in the subclinical apoplexy group compared with the acute apoplexy group. Headaches did resolve after surgical resection. The discrepancy between the apoplexy severity between the 2 cohorts in this study suggests that the authors followed a similar decision tree as described previously. A relevant decision tree is shown in **Fig. 3**.

NATURAL HISTORY BEFORE APOPLEXY

In a small but prospective natural history study, Arita and colleagues[24] demonstrated that 9.5% of patients with pituitary macroadenomas developed pituitary apoplexy at 5-year follow-up. This finding has led to class 3 evidence supporting elective resection of asymptomatic nonfunctional pituitary macroadenomas.[33] Retrospective studies have investigated risk factors for apoplexy in patients with known pituitary adenomas, with anticoagulation (Moller-Goede and colleagues[34]) and large fluid shifts occurring during cardiothoracic operations (Pliam and colleagues[35]) suggested to be risk factors. Others have also found that many pituitary apoplexy patients have reduced access to medical care before their apoplexy, and, in retrospect, endorse symptoms that could have led to adenomas diagnosis had these symptoms been evaluated by a medical provider.[36]

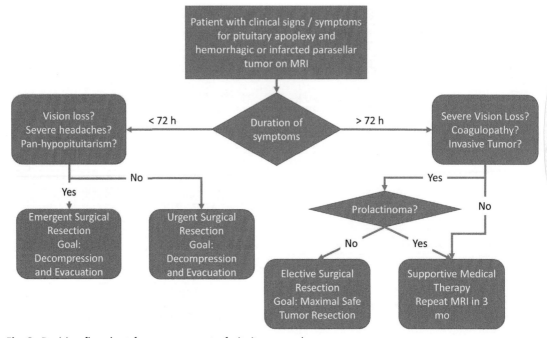

Fig. 3. Decision flowchart for management of pituitary apoplexy.

SUMMARY

Pituitary apoplexy is a clinical diagnosis with a combination of severe headaches, vision loss, double vision, and/or hypopituitarism, along with a hemorrhagic or infarcted pituitary lesion. Treatment is predicated upon symptom severity and timing. Urgent or emergent surgical resection remains the mainstay for acute pituitary apoplexy, especially with vision loss.

REFERENCES

1. Fernandez A, Karavitaki N, Wass JA. Prevalence of pituitary adenomas: a community-based, cross-sectional study in Banbury (Oxfordshire, UK). Clin Endocrinol 2010;72(3):377–82.
2. Raappana A, Koivukangas J, Ebeling T, et al. Incidence of pituitary adenomas in Northern Finland in 1992–2007. J Clin Endocrinol Metab 2010;95(9):4268–75.
3. Semple P, Webb M, de Villiers J, et al. Pituitary apoplexy. Neurosurgery 2005;56(1):65.
4. Briet C, Salenave S, Bonneville J, et al. Pituitary apoplexy. Endocr Rev 2015;36(6):622.
5. Biousse V, Newman N, Oyesiku N. Precipitating factors in pituitary apoplexy. J Neurol Neurosurg Psychiatry 2001;71(4):542.
6. Clarke J, Johnston S, Farrant M, et al. External validation of the ICH score. Neurocrit Care 2004;1(1):53.
7. McLaughlin N, Laws E, Oyesiku N, et al. Pituitary centers of excellence. Neurosurgery 2012;71(5):916.
8. Danesh-Meyer H, Wong A, Papchenko T, et al. Optical coherence tomography predicts visual outcome for pituitary tumors. J Clin Neurosci 2015;22(7):1098.
9. Murray JS, Jayarajasingh R, Perros P. Lesson of the week: deterioration of symptoms after start of thyroid hormone replacement. BMJ 2001;323(7308):332.
10. Bordo G, Kelly K, McLaughlin N, et al. Sellar masses that present with severe hyponatremia. Endocr Pract 2014;20(11):1178.
11. Laureno R. Central pontine myelinolysis following rapid correction of hyponatremia. Ann Neurol 1983;13(3):232.
12. Asa SL, Ezzat S, Kelly DF, et al. Hypothalamic vasopressin-producing tumors. Am J Surg Pathol 2019;43(2):251–60.
13. Hage R, Eshraghi SR, Oyesiku NM, et al. Third, fourth, and sixth cranial nerve palsies in pituitary apoplexy. World Neurosurg 2016;94:447.
14. Brisman M, Katz G, Post K. Symptoms of pituitary apoplexy rapidly reversed with bromocriptine. Case report. J Neurosurg 1996;85(6):1153.
15. Gondim J, de Albuquerque L, Almeida J, et al. Endoscopic endonasal surgery for treatment of pituitary apoplexy: 16 years of experience in a specialized pituitary center. World Neurosurg 2017;108:137.
16. Rutkowski M, Kunwar S, Blevins L, et al. Surgical intervention for pituitary apoplexy: an analysis of functional outcomes. J Neurosurg 2018;129(2):417.

17. Marcet P, Paluzzi J, Morrison A, et al. Endocrine outcomes of trans-sphenoidal surgery for pituitary apoplexy versus elective surgery for pituitary adenoma. Endocr Pract 2019;25(4):353–60.

18. Liu Z, Chang C, Pai P, et al. Clinical features and surgical outcome of clinical and subclinical pituitary apoplexy. J Clin Neurosci 2010;17(6):694.

19. Conger AR, Zhao F, Wang X, et al. Evolution of the graded repair of cerebrospinal fluid leaks and skull base defects in endonasal endoscopic tumor surgery: trends in repair failure and meningitis rates in 509 patients. J Neurol Surg B Skull Base 2018; 79(S 01):A203.

20. Semple P, Jane J, Lopes M, et al. Pituitary apoplexy: correlation between magnetic resonance imaging and histopathological results. J Neurosurg 2008; 108(5):909.

21. Jeffcoate W, Birch C. Apoplexy in small pituitary tumours. J Neurol Neurosurg Psychiatry 1986;49(9): 1077.

22. Pelkonen R, Kuusisto A, Salmi J, et al. Pituitary function after pituitary apoplexy. Am J Med 1978;65(5): 773.

23. Sibal L, Ball S, Connolly V, et al. Pituitary apoplexy: a review of clinical presentation, management and outcome in 45 cases. Pituitary 2004;7(3):157.

24. Arita K, Tominaga A, Sugiyama K, et al. Natural course of incidentally found nonfunctioning pituitary adenoma, with special reference to pituitary apoplexy during follow-up examination. J Neurosurg 2006;104(6):884.

25. Ayuk J, McGregor E, Mitchell R, et al. Acute management of pituitary apoplexy–surgery or conservative management? Clin Endocrinol 2004;61(6):747.

26. Bonicki W, Kasperlik-Załuska A, Koszewski W, et al. Pituitary apoplexy: endocrine, surgical and oncological emergency. Incidence, clinical course and treatment with reference to 799 cases of pituitary adenomas. Acta Neurochir 1993;120(3–4):118.

27. Gruber A, Clayton J, Kumar S, et al. Pituitary apoplexy: retrospective review of 30 patients–is surgical intervention always necessary? Br J Neurosurg 2006;20(6):379.

28. Leyer C, Castinetti F, Morange I, et al. A conservative management is preferable in milder forms of pituitary tumor apoplexy. J Endocrinol Invest 2011;34(7):502.

29. Maccagnan P, Macedo C, Kayath M, et al. Conservative management of pituitary apoplexy: a prospective study. J Clin Endocrinol Metab 1995; 80(7):2190.

30. Tu M, Lu Q, Zhu P, et al. Surgical versus non-surgical treatment for pituitary apoplexy: a systematic review and meta-analysis. J Neurol Sci 2016;370:258–62.

31. Rajasekaran S, Vanderpump M, Baldeweg S, et al. UK guidelines for the management of pituitary apoplexy. Clin Endocrinol 2011;74(1):9.

32. Bujawansa S, Thondam S, Steele C, et al. Presentation, management and outcomes in acute pituitary apoplexy: a large single-centre experience from the United Kingdom. Clin Endocrinol 2014; 80(3):419.

33. Aghi M, Chen C, Fleseriu M, et al. Congress of neurological surgeons systematic review and evidence-based guidelines on the management of patients with nonfunctioning pituitary adenomas: executive summary. Neurosurgery 2016;79(4):521.

34. Möller-Goede D, Brändle M, Landau K, et al. Pituitary apoplexy: re evaluation of risk factors for bleeding into pituitary adenomas and impact on outcome. Eur J Endocrinol 2011;164(1):37.

35. Pliam M, Cohen M, Cheng L, et al. Pituitary adenomas complicating cardiac surgery: summary and review of 11 cases. J Card Surg 1995;10(2):125.

36. Jahangiri A, Clark A, Han S, et al. Socioeconomic factors associated with pituitary apoplexy. J Neurosurg 2013;119(6):1432.

Surgery for Pediatric Pituitary Adenomas

Alexandria C. Marino, MD, PhD, Davis G. Taylor, MD, Bhargav Desai, MD,
John A. Jane Jr, MD*

KEYWORDS

- Pituitary adenomas • Pediatric • Cushing disease • Growth hormone • ACTH • Prolactinoma
- Transsphenoidal

KEY POINTS

- Pediatric pituitary adenomas are rare but are important to diagnose because of their potential implications on growth and development.
- Many pediatric pituitary tumors are managed with resection through a transsphenoidal approach.
- Variations in sphenoid pneumatization and anatomic measurements in pediatric patients warrant careful examination of preoperative imaging and use of intraoperative adjuncts such as image guidance and Doppler.
- With appropriate planning, transsphenoidal resection of pediatric pituitary tumors leads to outcomes comparable with those in adult patients.

▶ Video content accompanies this article at http://www.neurosurgery.theclinics.com.

INTRODUCTION

Tumors of the pituitary gland and sella region, although common in adulthood, are uncommon in children, constituting just 3% of all cranial lesions.[1–4] When present, pediatric sellar lesions are more likely to represent craniopharyngiomas or Rathke cleft cysts than adenomas. Because of varying types of tumors that occur in children and the effects that pituitary tumors may have on the developing hypothalamic-pituitary axis in prepubescent children, the presentation of pituitary lesions can be different in children than in adults.[5] This article describes the clinical differences between adult and pediatric patients presenting with pituitary adenomas and emphasizes the surgical considerations for pediatric sellar lesions.[3,4]

SYMPTOMS AND DIAGNOSTIC TESTING

Adenomas cause symptoms through hypersecretion or compression effects on nearby structures. This process occurs in both pediatric and adult populations, but symptoms may manifest differently in children. Endocrine disruptions in children caused by pituitary suppression or hypersecretion are especially concerning because of their potential effects on growth, development, and puberty. Further, the demographics of tumor subtypes are different among adults compared with children. In adults, nonfunctional adenomas are more common than functional tumors, and prolactinomas occur most frequently among hypersecreting adenomas.[1,6,7] In contrast, adrenocorticotropic hormone (ACTH)–secreting tumors are the most common tumor in children,

Disclosure: The authors have nothing to disclose.
Department of Neurological Surgery, University of Virginia Health Sciences Center, PO Box 800212, Charlottesville, VA 22908, USA
* Corresponding author.
E-mail address: jaj2k@virginia.edu

Neurosurg Clin N Am 30 (2019) 465–471
https://doi.org/10.1016/j.nec.2019.05.008

followed by prolactinomas, growth hormone (GH)—secreting adenomas, and nonfunctioning adenomas.[3,8,9] Within pediatric populations, ACTH-secreting tumors are overly represented in prepubescent children, whereas prolactinomas are more common after puberty.[3,8,9] Adenomas in children are also more likely to be functional hypersecreting tumors, because many nonfunctioning adenomas are slow growing and may not cause pituitary axis insufficiency or visual symptoms until the child is well into adulthood.[10] Although most pituitary adenomas in children are sporadic, they are more likely to occur as part of a congenital genetic condition such as Carney complex, McCune-Albright syndrome, multiple endocrine neoplasia type 1, or familial isolated pituitary adenomas.[3]

Work-up of children with suspected pituitary lesions is similar to that of adults. Children should receive thorough endocrine laboratory work-up, including thyroid-stimulating hormone/free T4, luteinizing hormone, follicle-stimulating hormone, testosterone in boys, prolactin, GH, insulinlike growth factor 1 (IGF-1), ACTH, and cortisol, as well as thin-cut, contrast-enhanced MRI through the sella. If visual field deficits are suspected, baseline ophthalmologic testing is warranted. In very young patients, genetic diseases such as MEN-1, McCune-Albright syndrome, Carney complex, and familial isolated pituitary adenomas should be considered.[3] In the pediatric population, plotting of height and weight growth charts should be performed. Although children with Cushing disease often experience growth arrest, children with GH adenomas experience accelerated growth. Once the diagnosis is confirmed, treatment should be planned by a multimodal team including at minimum endocrinology and neurosurgery. This article reviews the symptomatic presentation, diagnostic considerations, and medical management strategies specific to several of the most common adenoma subtypes.

Adrenocorticotropic Hormone–Secreting Adenoma (Cushing Disease)

ACTH-secreting adenomas in children can present with weight gain, glucose intolerance, and hypertension as in adults, but in particular with pubertal delay or growth arrest.[11] Growth retardation can be more severe in prepubertal patients. In contrast with adults, children are less likely to experience neurologic symptoms or muscle weakness.[3]

Proper diagnosis of Cushing disease is a multistep process. The initial evaluation centers on the confirmation of cortisol excess, which includes the low-dose dexamethasone suppression test,

the 24-hour urinary free cortisol, and the late-night salivary cortisol tests. Each of these tests has a similar rate of false-positives, and diagnosis should be confirmed with repeated testing. After Cushing syndrome is confirmed, random ACTH levels indicate whether the disease is ACTH dependent. If ACTH dependency is confirmed, suppression with a high-dose dexamethasone test can suggest a pituitary source. If positive, pituitary MRI is then appropriate. Pituitary MRI before biochemical evidence of a pituitary source may lead to misdiagnosis given the frequency of incidental findings on MRI. The pituitary MRI sequences should include VIBE (volumetric interpolated breath-hold examination) sequences because these have been shown to more reliably identify microadenomas. If negative, a dynamic MRI scan may be pursued. If MRI remains unrevealing, inferior petrosal sinus sampling should be considered to confirm a pituitary source.

Prolactinoma

Presenting symptoms in prolactinomas can vary depending on age, sexual maturity, and gender. Some children, especially boys, present with symptoms caused by mass effect. Prolactin secretion can lead to galactorrhea and amenorrhea in adolescent girls, although galactorrhea is less common than in adult women. Young female patients may present with primary rather than secondary amenorrhea.[12] Growth can also be delayed in children whose epiphyseal plates have not yet fused.[13] Prolactin levels greater than 200 ng/mL are diagnostic, and children with this finding should receive MRI. Small prolactinomas can yield prolactin levels from 30 to 200 ng/mL and, depending on symptoms, imaging may be warranted in these children. In the context of a macroadenoma (>1 cm) and moderately increased prolactin level (<200 ng/mL), a nonfunctioning adenoma causing stalk effect should be considered.[14] Even in children, the possibility of pregnancy should be evaluated as well as other causes of hyperprolactinemia, including medications and hypothyroidism. When questions regarding diagnosis between prolactinoma and nonfunctioning adenoma arise, a trial of dopamine agonist therapy may be appropriate. In almost all cases, only prolactinomas decrease in size with medical therapy.

Once confirmed, medical management is appropriate for pediatric prolactinomas. As in adults, pediatric patients with prolactinomas most often can be treated with dopamine agonists. At present, cabergoline is the preferred first-line therapy because of its efficacy and improved side effect profile, but cost considerations may make bromocriptine a reasonable choice.[15] Medical therapy effectively reduces serum prolactin levels and tumor size in 70% of patients with microadenomas and 90% of patients with macroadenomas.[16] Dopamine agonists seem to be well tolerated long term, but cabergoline has not been specifically studied in the pediatric population.[17] For most patients, medical therapy is suppressive and requires lifelong therapy. A small percentage of patients with small tumors may be able to discontinue medical therapy several years after achieving biochemical and radiographic remission. Although medical management is appropriate for most patients, those with noninvasive tumors may be offered surgical resection for the chance of a long-term remission and avoidance of long-term medical therapy. Although most patients respond to medical therapy, some prolactinomas are radiographically refractory to medical management and require surgical management.[18,19]

Growth Hormone–Secreting Adenoma

GH-secreting adenoma presentation can vary with age. In children whose epiphyseal plates have not yet fused, patients may present with gigantism. The associated rapid linear growth can cause children to reach heights and weights several standard deviations greater than their peers and expected heights based on parental measurement (**Fig. 1**).

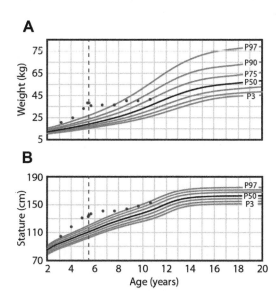

A

B

Fig. 1. Correction of abnormal growth with transsphenoidal surgery in a pediatric patient with gigantism attributable to a growth hormone–secreting pituitary adenomas. (*A*) Weight-for-age and (*B*) stature-for-age plots for a patient with gigantism treated with transsphenoidal surgery. Lines mark 3rd, 10th, 25th, 50th, 75th, 90th, and 97th percentiles; time of surgery is marked by vertical dashed line.

Patients with gigantism may also show increased organ size and soft tissue volume as well as systemic disease such as diabetes, hypertension, and heart failure.[20] Older children whose epiphyseal plates have already fused experience symptoms similar to those of adults with acromegaly; namely, enlarged lips, nose, tongue, hands, and feet, and obesity.[21] Laboratory work-up is notable for increased IGF-1 and a failure to reach a nadir GH level of less than 0.4 ng/mL during an oral glucose tolerance test. A random GH level cannot be used for diagnosis because GH levels are highly variable throughout the day.[22]

Medical therapy can be pursued in GH-secreting adenomas using dopamine agonists such as cabergoline, somatostatin receptor agonists, and/or the human GH receptor antagonist pegvisomant.[23] Patients with only modestly increased IGF-1 levels may respond to dopamine agonists; however, somatostatin agonists and pegvisomant are more likely to be chosen for patients who have greater increases in IGF-1 levels and symptoms.[22] Medical therapy is less effective in tumor volume reduction and is less often chosen for patients who present with chiasmal compression and visual deficits. Many practitioners suggest reserving medical therapy as a rescue treatment if surgery fails, and these medications are poorly studied in pediatric patients.[24]

MEDICAL AND SURGICAL THERAPIES

Surgery is the first-line treatment modality for patients with nonfunctioning macroadenomas, Cushing disease, and most GH-secreting tumors. Patients with prolactinomas that continue to grow despite medical management (radiographically refractory) or have persistently increased prolactin levels (biochemically refractory) warrant consideration of surgery. In addition, surgery is reasonable for those patients who are intolerant of medication therapy secondary to side effects or may not be able to succeed with long-term medication compliance. Resection is typically conducted via a microscopic or endoscopic transsphenoidal technique. The endoscopic technique is increasingly used with satisfactory outcomes and shorter hospital stays.[25–27]

The surgical approach for pediatric patients is comparable with that in adults, and has been previously described.[28] At our institution, we have begun using the endoscopic approach more often, although microscopic approaches may still be used.[29] Although variations are available, at our institution patients are placed in a beach-chair position and the head is flexed such that the bridge of the nose parallels the floor. The head is fixed in a

Mayfield head holder and a neuronavigation system is used. The head of the patient and the operating table is rotated toward the surgeon with the monitor placed directly in the surgeon's line of sight. When using an endoscope, an otorhinolaryngologist typically performs the initial approach to the sella and may create a nasoseptal flap to aid in closure and minimize the risk of a cerebrospinal fluid (CSF) leak, although a nasoseptal flap may be challenging to create in children less than 10 years of age because of their small septal area relative to typical skull base defects.[30–32] The bony anterior face of the sella is removed and the dura is opened with the intent of not traversing into the pituitary capsule or tumor (Video 1). When technically possible, resection taking advantage of the histologic pseudocapsule leads to high probability of total resection without a higher chance of new endocrinopathy.[33] Challenges presented by the smaller operative corridor in children can be partially overcome by tailoring the surgical approach. Although lateralization of the turbinates is preferred, as in adult patients, some otorhinolaryngologists prefer removal of some portion of the turbinates to create room. The posterior septectomy should be generous.[34] The smaller nares in pediatric patients may limit the surgeon's operative corridor and diminish the ability to maneuver within the pituitary fossa.[35] In addition, transsphenoidal surgery can be conducted via a sublabial approach, taking advantage of the width of the piriform aperture.

Once the sella is reached, there are important anatomic distinctions to consider in pediatric patients before approaching the pituitary, particularly with respect to the pneumatization of the sphenoid sinus. At birth, the sphenoid bone is usually solid. Pneumatization begins around the age of 2 years and continues until adolescence.[36,37] Pneumatization patterns can be defined as conchal, which denotes a solid sphenoid bone, or presellar, sellar, or postsellar (**Fig. 2**). In the case of a sellar or postsellar pneumatization pattern, as is most common in adults, only a thin layer of bone (or sometimes no bone) separates the sphenoid sinus from the sella or the adjacent critical structures such as the optic nerves, carotid arteries, and cavernous sinus. In well-pneumatized bone, the presence of bony landmarks and predictable septations often allows the surgeon to more readily identify the

opticocarotid cisterns and other sellar landmarks.[38–40] However, in children with little pneumatization, such as conchal pneumatization, it may be difficult to identify bony landmarks to aid the surgeon in the approach.[41] In these cases, safe surgical exposure requires drilling of the nonpneumatized bone (Video 2) and the aid of intraoperative Doppler or neuronavigation for the identification of the carotid arteries (see Video 1). With these precautions it is possible to resect pituitary adenomas even in the case of conchal pneumatization, although the difficulty of resection increases with the size of the lesion given the increased amount of bone that must be drilled away.[34,42]

Other anatomic measurements should be considered when planning transsphenoidal surgery in pediatric patients (**Fig. 3**). The intercarotid distance should be noted and planned for operatively.[43] When measured at the superior clivus, the intercarotid distance is adult sized by age 2 years; however, when measured at the cavernous sinus, studies conflict as to whether the intercarotid distance varies with age or not, with at least 1 group finding this distance to be smaller before age 7 years.[34,35,37] The piriform aperture, which serves as a limiting bony structure, is narrower in children less than 7 years old.[37] Other important measurements do not vary with age but do vary from measurements found in healthy children. Pediatric patients with skull base lesions have shorter naresellar and vomer-clivus distances, and smaller transsphenoidal angles, all of which are relevant to surgical planning.[34] These measurements should be examined on preoperative imaging to ensure that a desirable extent of resection is possible.

After surgery, patients should undergo routing monitoring for postoperative complications, such as diabetes insipidus, hypocortisolism, and CSF leaks. Patients should be discharged with appropriate endocrinology follow-up to continue monitoring for adrenal insufficiency, hypothyroidism, GH deficiency, or diabetes insipidus.

SURGICAL OUTCOMES AND COMPLICATIONS

Outcomes and complications for adults with pituitary adenomas have been extensively studied.

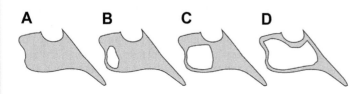

Fig. 2. Sphenoid pneumatization patterns. The sphenoid bone with (*A*) conchal, (*B*) presellar, (*C*) sellar, and (*D*) postsellar pneumatization patterns.

A **B** **C** **D**

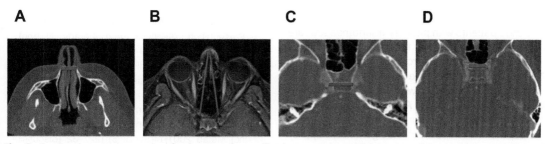

Fig. 3. Anatomic measurements of relevance for pediatric transsphenoidal surgery. (*A*) Axial bone-windowed computed tomography shows piriform aperture (*red line*). (*B*) Axial T1 postcontrast MRI shows transsphenoidal angle (*red lines*). Intercarotid distance (*red lines*) at the (*C*) superior clivus and (*D*) cavernous sinus; note the incomplete pneumatization of the sphenoid sinus.

Depending on the tumor type, 56% to 91% of adult patients with hypersecreting tumors experience endocrinological remission. In addition, 87% of patients can expect improvements in visual loss with surgery, and 27% of patients presenting with pituitary suppression experience return to normal function. The recurrence rate in adults is generally low when gross total resection is achieved, around 13% at 10 years.[44] Transient diabetes insipidus occurs in about 10% of patients and postoperative CSF leak generally remains less than 5%.[45]

The percentage of remission, recurrence, and incidence of complications is highly variable in the small pediatric case series that have been published; for example, recurrence has been reported to be as low as 8%[46] and as high as 70%.[47] The number of patients included in these individual studies is generally small and often includes patients cared for by a single surgeon; this makes variability in outcomes difficult to interpret. However, a recent meta-analysis of previously published surgical series as well as a separate retrospective study using a widely available pediatric inpatient database are both notable for including more than 800 pediatric patients. In a cohort of 831 pediatric patients that underwent transsphenoidal endoscopic resection of a pituitary lesion, diabetes insipidus (either transient or persistent) occurred in 30.4%, panhypopituitarism occurred in 10.2%, and CSF leak occurred in 2.3%.[48] A separate meta-analysis of pediatric case series published from 1978 to 2017 included 1284 pediatric patients and found that recurrence occurred in 35%, whereas complications of panhypopituitarism, chronic diabetes insipidus, and CSF leak occurred in 23%, 3%, and 4%, respectively.[49] These data are consistent with outcomes reported at our institution.[50] From these reports, it seems that transsphenoidal surgery in pediatric patients is safe and that gross total or subtotal resection with symptomatic improvement can be achieved in most patients. The most common postoperative complications of diabetes insipidus, hypopituitarism, and CSF leak occur at a rate comparable with to adult patients; this emphasizes the need for close postoperative laboratory monitoring with the involvement of an endocrinologist. Further study is needed to determine whether the higher recurrence rate in pediatric patients is a true effect or is attributable to variations in length of follow-up.

MANAGEMENT OF RESIDUAL AND RECURRENCE

Several patients are left with residual tumor or experience recurrence after resection. Residual tumors in the case of prolactinomas and GH-secreting tumors can be managed medically, and data in adults suggest that medically refractory patients may become responsive after surgical debulking.[51,52] Some surgeons elect to proceed with adjuvant gamma knife radiosurgery for residual tumors and this is particularly considered for Cushing disease with invasion of the cavernous sinus.[53] Recurrences after apparent total resection of a nonfunctioning adenoma may be managed with further surgery or with radiosurgery. Although rarely studied in the pediatric population, 75% of adult patients with nonfunctioning adenomas that recurred after surgery experienced tumor shrinkage when treated with gamma knife radiosurgery,[54] and pediatric patients with Cushing disease that recurred can also experience remission with radiotherapy.[55] Recurrences may be especially problematic in pediatric patients given their anticipated long follow-up; in addition, some controversy exists as to what constitutes an acceptable risk from gamma knife radiosurgery in pediatric patients, with some clinicians limiting gamma knife to older children.[56] Further study is warranted to determine the best course for recurrence in pediatric patients.

SUMMARY

Pediatric patients with pituitary adenomas are rare but important childhood tumors with significant implications on normal growth and development. Neurosurgeons should be aware of the ways in which symptoms vary between adults and children with pituitary adenomas. A significant number of these tumors warrant surgical resection, and a transsphenoidal approach is generally appropriate. Given the variations in sphenoid pneumatization and anatomic measurements particular to children, careful examination of preoperative imaging and intraoperative adjuncts, such as image guidance and Doppler, may be helpful. With these steps, resection of pediatric pituitary adenomas can be safely undertaken, with complication rates comparable with those seen in adult patients.

SUPPLEMENTARY DATA

Supplementary data related to this article can be found online at https://doi.org/10.1016/j.nec.2019.05.008.

REFERENCES

1. Ezzat S, Asa SL, Couldwell WT, et al. The prevalence of pituitary adenomas: a systematic review. Cancer 2004;101(3):613–9.
2. Al-Dahmani K, Mohammad S, Imran F, et al. Sellar masses: an epidemiological study. Can J Neurol Sci 2016;43(2):291–7.
3. Keil MF, Stratakis CA. Pituitary tumors in childhood: update of diagnosis, treatment and molecular genetics. Expert Rev Neurother 2008;8(4):563–74.
4. Laws ER, Scheithauer BW, Groover RV. Pituitary adenomas in childhood and adolescence. Prog Exp Tumor Res 1987;30:359–61.
5. Lafferty AR, Chrousos GP. Pituitary tumors in children and adolescents. J Clin Endocrinol Metab 1999;84(12):4317–23.
6. Daly AF, Rixhon M, Adam C, et al. High prevalence of pituitary adenomas: a cross-sectional study in the province of Liege, Belgium. J Clin Endocrinol Metab 2006;91(12):4769–75.
7. Jagannathan J, Kanter AS, Sheehan JP, et al. Benign brain tumors: sellar/parasellar tumors. Neurol Clin 2007;25(4):1231–49, xi.
8. Mehrazin M. Pituitary tumors in children: clinical analysis of 21 cases. Childs Nerv Syst 2007;23(4): 391–8.
9. Pandey P, Ojha BK, Mahapatra AK. Pediatric pituitary adenoma: a series of 42 patients. J Clin Neurosci 2005;12(2):124–7.
10. Krajewski KL, Rotermund R, Flitsch J. Pituitary adenomas in children and young adults. Childs Nerv Syst 2018;34(9):1691–6.
11. Magiakou MA, Mastorakos G, Oldfield EH, et al. Cushing's syndrome in children and adolescents. Presentation, diagnosis, and therapy. N Engl J Med 1994;331(10):629–36.
12. Fideleff HL, Boquete HR, Suarez MG, et al. Prolactinoma in children and adolescents. Horm Res 2009; 72(4):197–205.
13. Duntas LH. Prolactinomas in children and adolescents–consequences in adult life. J Pediatr Endocrinol Metab 2001;14(Suppl 5):1227–32 [discussion: 1261–2].
14. Mehmed S, Polonsky K, Larsen P, et al. Pituitary masses and tumors. In: Williams textbook of endocrinology. 13th edition. Philadelphia: Elsevier; 2016. p. 232–99.
15. Webster J, Piscitelli G, Polli A, et al. A comparison of cabergoline and bromocriptine in the treatment of hyperprolactinemic amenorrhea. Cabergoline Comparative Study Group. N Engl J Med 1994;331(14):904–9.
16. Molitch ME, Elton RL, Blackwell RE, et al. Bromocriptine as primary therapy for prolactin-secreting macroadenomas: results of a prospective multicenter study. J Clin Endocrinol Metab 1985;60(4):698–705.
17. Schlechte JA. Long-term management of prolactinomas. J Clin Endocrinol Metab 2007;92(8):2861–5.
18. Spinks JJ, Ryan FJ. Cabergoline resistance in pediatric prolactinomas. J Pediatr Hematol Oncol 2009; 31(5):377–9.
19. Vroonen L, Jaffrain-Rea ML, Petrossians P, et al. Prolactinomas resistant to standard doses of cabergoline: a multicenter study of 92 patients. Eur J Endocrinol 2012;167(5):651–62.
20. Guaraldi F, Storr HL, Ghizzoni L, et al. Paediatric pituitary adenomas: a decade of change. Horm Res Paediatr 2014;81(3):145–55.
21. Laws ER Jr, Scheithauer BW, Carpenter S, et al. The pathogenesis of acromegaly. Clinical and immunocytochemical analysis in 75 patients. J Neurosurg 1985;63(1):35–8.
22. Katznelson L, Laws ER Jr, Melmed S, et al. Acromegaly: an endocrine society clinical practice guideline. J Clin Endocrinol Metab 2014;99(11):3933–51.
23. Feenstra J, de Herder WW, ten Have SM, et al. Combined therapy with somatostatin analogues and weekly pegvisomant in active acromegaly. Lancet 2005;365(9471):1644–6.
24. Bush ZM, Vance ML. Management of acromegaly: is there a role for primary medical therapy? Rev Endocr Metab Disord 2008;9(1):83–94.
25. Singh H, Essayed WI, Cohen-Gadol A, et al. Resection of pituitary tumors: endoscopic versus microscopic. J Neurooncol 2016;130(2):309–17.
26. Asemota AO, Ishii M, Brem H, et al. Comparison of complications, trends, and costs in endoscopic vs microscopic pituitary surgery: analysis from a US Health Claims Database. Neurosurgery 2017;81(3): 458–72.

27. Rolston JD, Han SJ, Aghi MK. Nationwide shift from microscopic to endoscopic transsphenoidal pituitary surgery. Pituitary 2016;19(3):248–50.

28. Jane JA Jr, Thapar K, Kaptain GJ, et al. Pituitary surgery: transsphenoidal approach. Neurosurgery 2002;51(2):435–42 [discussion: 442–4].

29. Chen CJ, Ironside N, Pomeraniec IJ, et al. Microsurgical versus endoscopic transsphenoidal resection for acromegaly: a systematic review of outcomes and complications. Acta Neurochir (Wien) 2017; 159(11):2193–207.

30. Hadad G, Bassagasteguy L, Carrau RL, et al. A novel reconstructive technique after endoscopic expanded endonasal approaches: vascular pedicle nasoseptal flap. Laryngoscope 2006;116(10):1882–6.

31. Ghosh A, Hatten K, Learned KO, et al. Pediatric nasoseptal flap reconstruction for suprasellar approaches. Laryngoscope 2015;125(11):2451–6.

32. Shah RN, Surowitz JB, Patel MR, et al. Endoscopic pedicled nasoseptal flap reconstruction for pediatric skull base defects. Laryngoscope 2009;119(6): 1067–75.

33. Taylor DG, Jane JA, Oldfield EH. Resection of pituitary macroadenomas via the pseudocapsule along the posterior tumor margin: a cohort study and technical note. J Neurosurg 2018;128(2):422–8.

34. Banu MA, Rathman A, Patel KS, et al. Corridor-based endonasal endoscopic surgery for pediatric skull base pathology with detailed radioanatomic measurements. Neurosurgery 2014;10(Suppl 2): 273–93 [discussion: 293].

35. Tatreau JR, Patel MR, Shah RN, et al. Anatomical limitations for endoscopic endonasal skull base surgery in pediatric patients. Laryngoscope 2010; 120(Suppl 4):S229.

36. Gruber DP, Brockmeyer D. Pediatric skull base surgery. 1. Embryology and developmental anatomy. Pediatr Neurosurg 2003;38(1):2–8.

37. Tatreau JR, Patel MR, Shah RN, et al. Anatomical considerations for endoscopic endonasal skull base surgery in pediatric patients. Laryngoscope 2010;120(9):1730–7.

38. Batra PS, Citardi MJ, Gallivan RP, et al. Software-enabled computed tomography analysis of the carotid artery and sphenoid sinus pneumatization patterns. Am J Rhinol 2004;18(4):203–8.

39. Guldner C, Pistorius SM, Diogo I, et al. Analysis of pneumatization and neurovascular structures of the sphenoid sinus using cone-beam tomography (CBT). Acta Radiol 2012;53(2):214–9.

40. Tomovic S, Esmaeili A, Chan NJ, et al. High-resolution computed tomography analysis of variations of the sphenoid sinus. J Neurol Surg B Skull Base 2013;74(2):82–90.

41. Kuan EC, Kaufman AC, Lerner D, et al. Lack of sphenoid pneumatization does not affect

42. Hamid O, El Fiky L, Hassan O, et al. Anatomic variations of the sphenoid sinus and their impact on trans-sphenoid pituitary surgery. Skull Base 2008; 18(1):9–15.

43. Renn WH, Rhoton AL Jr. Microsurgical anatomy of the sellar region. J Neurosurg 1975;43(3):288–98.

44. Jane JA Jr, Laws ER Jr. The surgical management of pituitary adenomas in a series of 3,093 patients. J Am Coll Surg 2001;193(6):651–9.

45. Barker FG 2nd, Klibanski A, Swearingen B. Transsphenoidal surgery for pituitary tumors in the United States, 1996-2000: mortality, morbidity, and the effects of hospital and surgeon volume. J Clin Endocrinol Metab 2003;88(10):4709–19.

46. Richmond IL, Wilson CB. Pituitary adenomas in childhood and adolescence. J Neurosurg 1978; 49(2):163–8.

47. Cannavo S, Venturino M, Curto L, et al. Clinical presentation and outcome of pituitary adenomas in teenagers. Clin Endocrinol (Oxf) 2003;58(4):519–27.

48. Hanba C, Svider PF, Shkoukani MA, et al. Pediatric pituitary resection: characterizing surgical approaches and complications. Int Forum Allergy Rhinol 2017;7(1):72–9.

49. Perry A, Graffeo CS, Marcellino C, et al. Pediatric pituitary adenoma: case series, review of the literature, and a skull base treatment paradigm. J Neurol Surg B Skull Base 2018;79(1):91–114.

50. Kanter AS, Diallo AO, Jane JA Jr, et al. Single-center experience with pediatric Cushing's disease. J Neurosurg 2005;103(5 Suppl):413–20.

51. Hamilton DK, Vance ML, Boulos PT, et al. Surgical outcomes in hyporesponsive prolactinomas: analysis of patients with resistance or intolerance to dopamine agonists. Pituitary 2005;8(1):53–60.

52. Schwyzer L, Starke RM, Jane JA Jr, et al. Percent reduction of growth hormone levels correlates closely with percent resected tumor volume in acromegaly. J Neurosurg 2015;122(4):798–802.

53. Lonser RR, Ksendzovsky A, Wind JJ, et al. Prospective evaluation of the characteristics and incidence of adenoma-associated dural invasion in Cushing disease. J Neurosurg 2012;116(2):272–9.

54. Gopalan R, Schlesinger D, Vance ML, et al. Long-term outcomes after Gamma Knife radiosurgery for patients with a nonfunctioning pituitary adenoma. Neurosurgery 2011;69(2):284–93.

55. Acharya SV, Gopal RA, Goerge J, et al. Radiotherapy in paediatric Cushing's disease: efficacy and long term follow up of pituitary function. Pituitary 2010;13(4):293–7.

56. Murphy ES, Chao ST, Angelov L, et al. Radiosurgery for pediatric brain tumors. Pediatr Blood Cancer 2016;63(3):398–405.

Management of Nonfunctioning Recurrent Pituitary Adenomas

Christopher J. Farrell, MD[a,*], Tomas Garzon-Muvdi[a], Judd H. Fastenberg[b],
Gurston G. Nyquist[h], Mindy R. Rabinowitz[b], Marc R. Rosen[b],
James J. Evans[a]

KEYWORDS

- Recurrent pituitary tumor • KNOSP grade • Transsphenoidal surgery • Pituitary adenomas

KEY POINTS

- Pituitary adenomas have a high rate of progression following subtotal resection and recurrence after radiographic complete resection.
- Repeat transsphenoidal surgery for recurrent tumors is associated with reduced extent of resection compared with initial surgery and modestly increased risks of complications including endocrinopathy, cerebrospinal fluid leak, and visual worsening.
- Indications for repeat surgery include obtaining complete removal of recurrent tumors that are considered to be safely accessible, inducing endocrine remission for functional adenomas, relieving neurologic symptoms secondary to compression, and reducing the risks of stereotactic radiosurgery (SRS) by providing tumor clearance from radiation-sensitive structures such as the optic chiasm.
- SRS or fractionated stereotactic radiotherapy are safe and effective forms of radiation therapy for achieving long-term tumor control of recurrent pituitary adenomas.

INTRODUCTION

Pituitary adenomas account for approximately 10% to 20% of primary intracranial tumors.[1,2] Although these tumors are typically benign and slow growing, complete surgical resection is not always achievable and 50% to 60% of adenomas continue to progress after subtotal resection. The extent of resection at the time of primary surgical intervention depends highly on multiple factors including tumor size, consistency, dural invasion, and parasellar and suprasellar extension.[3,4] Even after apparent gross total resection, tumor recurrence may occur in up to 30% of cases with long-term follow-up.[5–9] Treatment options for recurrent pituitary adenomas include observation with serial neuroimaging, repeat surgical intervention via either the transsphenoidal or transcranial route, stereotactic radiosurgery, fractionated radiotherapy, and systemic medical therapy. There are few prospective studies available to guide treatment decisions for patients with recurrent pituitary adenomas, and numerous questions remain unanswered including the indications for repeat surgery and the type of surgery that should be performed, as well as the optimal timing, dose, and fractionation schedule for radiation therapy. This review provides an overview of the various treatment options for recurrent or progressive pituitary adenomas and discusses the authors' own experience with these challenging tumors.

Disclosure Statement: The authors have nothing to disclose.
[a] Department of Neurological Surgery, Thomas Jefferson University Hospital, Philadelphia, PA, USA;
[b] Department of Otolaryngology, Head and Neck Surgery, Thomas Jefferson University Hospital, Philadelphia, PA, USA
* Corresponding author. 909 Walnut Street 2nd Floor, Philadelphia, PA 19016.
E-mail address: christopher.farrell@jefferson.edu

NATURAL HISTORY OF PREVIOUSLY RESECTED PITUITARY ADENOMAS

Over the last several decades, there have been tremendous advances in the surgical techniques and technologies for pituitary adenomas; however, curative surgical resection remains difficult even in the hands of the most experienced surgeons. Progression rates after subtotal resection of pituitary adenomas are extremely high and recurrence rates following gross total resection increase with long-term follow-up. Traditionally, pituitary adenomas have been divided into either "functional" tumors that secrete pituitary hormones leading to an endocrinologic clinical syndrome or "nonfunctional" tumors that do not secrete pituitary hormones. Careful studies of nonfunctional pituitary adenomas (NFPAs), however, have revealed that many of these tumors do actually produce pituitary hormones, and the most recent fourth edition of the World Health Organization (WHO) classification of tumors of the pituitary gland has shifted from a hormone-producing classification to a pituitary adenohypophyseal cell-lineage designation based on hormone content, immunohistochemical features, and pituitary-specific transcription factors.[10,11] The new classification system also recognizes the importance of increased mitotic count, high Ki-67 proliferative index (>3%), and tumor invasion as pathologic markers of clinically aggressive adenomas with an increased risk of relapse and resistance to standard therapies. In addition, several subtypes of pituitary neuroendocrine tumors with a high probability of recurrence have been defined including silent corticotroph adenomas, sparsely granulated somatotroph adenomas, lactotroph adenomas in men, Crooke cell adenoma, and plurihormonal Pit-1-positive adenomas. This new pathologic classification should enable more accurate tumor subtyping and may allow improved prediction of aggressive clinical behavior to better assess and guide therapies in the setting of tumor recurrence.

SURGICAL TREATMENT OF RECURRENT PITUITARY ADENOMAS

Repeat surgery for pituitary adenomas is more difficult than primary surgery and is associated with lower rates of complete resection and endocrine remission as well as modestly increased complications.[12,13] In addition to the disruption or distortion of normal anatomic landmarks and the presence of scarring from the initial surgery that make repeat surgery more difficult, recurrent pituitary adenomas tend to be more invasive and more fibrous in consistency. As for most intracranial tumors, improved transsphenoidal pituitary surgery outcomes are correlated with increased hospital volume and surgeon volume.[14] In recognition of these challenges, before undertaking repeat surgery the authors advocate for a clear definition of the goals of surgery for each individual patient, a realistic assessment of the risks, anticipated extent of resection, hormonal and visual outcomes associated with the intervention, and an understanding of the surgical techniques and adjuncts that will allow for safer and more efficacious revision surgery.

The most common indications for repeat surgical intervention for recurrent NFPAs are to achieve complete removal of residual or progressive tumors that are considered to be safely accessible, relieve neurologic symptoms secondary to optic apparatus and cranial nerve compression or prevent impending symptoms, and to reduce the risk of other therapies, namely, stereotactic radiosurgery, by providing tumor debulking and clearance from radiation-sensitive structures such as the optic chiasm. Aggressive repeat surgery may also be necessary for tumors that have progressed despite prior radiation therapy or to achieve hormonal remission or improved endocrine control for functional adenomas. The decision to proceed with revision surgery often follows multidisciplinary consultation with radiation oncology, endocrinology, neuroradiology, and otolaryngology.

Surgery for recurrent pituitary adenomas is performed via either a transsphenoidal or transcranial route. Recently, a trend has emerged toward increased use of the endoscopic transsphenoidal approach, and several studies have reported on extent of adenoma resection, hormonal remission rates, and complications comparing the endoscopic and microscopic approaches.[15–20] Advantages of the endoscopic approach include the improved field of view with ability to use angled endoscopes and directly visualize the tumor interface with the normal pituitary gland and surrounding neurovascular structures, as well as the ability to perform bimanual dissection. In addition, the endoscopic approach allows for extended bony removal to access the suprasellar, parasellar, and clival regions if necessary. Despite these advantages in visualization and access, surgical outcomes using the endoscopic approach have not been definitively proved to be superior to those achieved with the microscopic approach for either primary or revision transsphenoidal surgery.[7,21,22] A recent meta-analysis performed by Esquenazi and colleagues[23] comparing endoscopic endonasal with microscopic transsphenoidal surgery for recurrent and progressive pituitary adenomas included 21 studies with 292 patients in the endoscopic group and 648 patients in the microscopic group. The pooled analysis revealed a gross total resection (GTR) of 53.5% for the endoscopic approach compared with 46.6% for the microscopic approach. Endocrinologic remission rates for functional adenomas were also increased in the endoscopic group, reported at 53.0% versus 46.7% of patients, respectively. Complication rates were slightly increased in the endoscopic group including postoperative cerebrospinal fluid (CSF) leak (4.4% vs 2.1%) and pituitary insufficiency (7.9% vs 5.2%), possibly related to more aggressive surgical resection. Interpretation of the results yielded by this meta-analysis is limited by the retrospective nature of the included studies and significant differences in adenoma size, biology (functional vs NFPA), type (residual vs recurrent), and cavernous sinus invasion between the 2 groups.

Several other large studies have reported on surgical outcomes following secondary transsphenoidal surgery, with improved results demonstrated for recurrent tumors compared with those with residual tumor and for NFPAs compared with functional adenomas. A meta-analysis performed by Heringer and colleagues[21] provided analysis of data pooled by tumor type for repeat surgical intervention. Overall remission rates for growth hormone–secreting tumors was 44.5% while remission rates for corticotropin hormone–secreting tumors was 55.5%. For NFPAs, a GTR rate of 76% (range 43%–93%) was reported. We (ie, the authors' group at Thomas Jefferson University) previously reported our outcomes using the endoscopic endonasal transsphenoidal approach for recurrent pituitary adenomas.[24] An overall GTR of 52% was observed with the extent of resection significantly correlated with Knosp grade cavernous sinus invasion, tumor size, and whether the initial surgery had been performed via either an endoscopic or microscopic transsphenoidal approach. Interestingly a GTR of 73% was achieved for patients previously operated on by the microscopic approach, compared with 35% for the endoscopic approach. Our impression, which has been shared by other highly experienced groups, is that inadequate exposure and reduced viewing angles provided by the microscopic approach may have been the primary determinant of subtotal resection during the initial transsphenoidal surgery.[3,6,25]

Preoperative and intraoperative considerations for revision surgery differ from those of primary transsphenoidal surgery. Before revision surgery, it is important to obtain as detailed information as possible from the initial surgery including the extent of bony removal, type of dural reconstruction performed, presence of any implants (eg, metallic mesh, cement) or packing materials (adipose graft), and any vascular complications. Knowledge of whether an intraoperative CSF leak was encountered during the initial surgery is also valuable because it predicts the likelihood of encountering a subsequent leak and potential need for a more extensive sellar reconstruction. Although cavernous sinus invasion can often be predicted radiographically, definitive assessment of invasion is determined intraoperatively and strongly correlates with extent of resection. Similarly, knowledge of dural invasion at the time of the initial surgery is important because resection of this involved dura should be performed in the setting of aggressive adenomas. Thorough reassessment of pituitary hormonal function should also be performed to detect previously undetected hormonal insufficiencies that will require replacement therapy and obtain baseline levels for determining endocrine remission for functional adenomas. In addition, as emphasized in the new WHO pituitary classification scheme, previously considered NFPAs may produce pituitary hormones, and transformation of silent corticotropic adenomas to functioning corticotropin-secreting adenomas has been reported in up to 9% of cases.[26]

The incidence of postoperative CSF leak is also increased with revision transsphenoidal surgery, and preoperative assessment of the viability of potential reconstruction options by careful preoperative sinonasal examination cannot be overstated in the revision setting. Prior transsphenoidal approaches often involve removal of tissues and destruction of key vascular structures. For example, expanded sphenoid openings may involve damage to the nasoseptal branch of the sphenopalatine artery and prevent use of the nasoseptal flap (NSF) for sellar reconstruction. A large posterior septectomy or septal perforation may also limit the amount of septal tissue available and render the NSF useless. Similarly, middle or inferior turbinectomy precludes the use of these tissues as rescue-flap options during reconstruction. Scarring near the sphenoid os or between the septal flaps may also make the vascular pedicle to the NSF tentative and elevation of the flap difficult.[19] We typically find that raising the NSF is easier on the side with less scarring. In our experience, a pedicled NSF is rarely necessary for cranial base repair during the initial standard transsphenoidal surgery for pituitary adenomas; however, owing to the potential for recurrence and need for subsequent revision surgery, we have previously described several tailored approaches that allow for unilateral preservation of the NSF.[27] Most frequently the "1.5 approach" is used, which involves an ipsilateral wide sphenoidotomy ("1") on the working instrument side with a limited contralateral sphenoidotomy superior to the sphenoid os ("0.5") on the endoscope side, which preserves the sphenopalatine artery pedicle to the NSF (**Fig. 1**). Additional use of an NSF at the time of initial surgery does not necessarily prohibit its reuse. Zanation and colleagues[28] demonstrated the ability to take down and reuse the NSF in both staged and revision cases with a high success rate and minimal additional nasal morbidity. In cases where a high-flow intraoperative CSF leak may be expected and preoperative sinonasal examination reveals absence of a viable NSF for reconstruction, additional rescue options need to be considered including reliance on nonvascularized reconstruction materials, CSF diversion via lumbar drainage, or harvest of a secondary pedicled flap such as a turbinate flap or tunneled temporoparietal fascia or pericranial flap.[29] Alternatively in these difficult cases a transcranial route may be preferable, especially for tumors that demonstrate significant intracranial extension lateral to the cavernous sinuses into the middle fossa or encase the arteries of the circle of Willis.[30]

Intraoperative considerations also differ between primary and revision transsphenoidal surgery. As stated previously, suboptimal exposure during the initial transsphenoidal surgery is often a contributing factor to subtotal resection (**Fig. 2**). During revision surgery, achieving a wide exposure is critical to opening up multiple surgical corridors for resection. During endoscopic endonasal transsphenoidal revision surgery, we perform a large sphenoidotomy with removal of any obstructing sphenoid bony septations. This provides adequate working room for the endoscope and dissection instruments and sufficient surgical exposure to allow for resection of tumors that extend laterally.[31] In revision surgery, surgical landmarks are often disrupted or distorted, and midline orientation may not be obvious. As such, neuronavigation with computed tomography (CT) and MRI is used for all revision surgeries with frequent confirmation of neuronavigation accuracy throughout the procedure using intact landmarks. Additional bony removal should be tailored based on the site of recurrence and extension. As a general principle, bony removal should be wider for revision surgery than primary surgery, where the tumors are often softer and more easily resectable. We routinely extend the sellar bony opening just beyond the medial walls of the cavernous sinuses, which allows for a maximally wide dural opening and potential extracapsular dissection of the tumor from the cavernous sinuses.[32] Internal debulking of recurrent pituitary adenomas is often more difficult because of the presence of extensive scar tissue within the sella from the prior resection as well as the often more fibrous consistency of the adenomas that have frequently contributed to the initial subtotal resection. Adequate tumor debulking for these firm tumors often requires sharp dissection or use of ultrasonic aspiration devices, or side-cutting rotatable microdebriders. Given the potential for vascular complications with these devices, we recommend use of

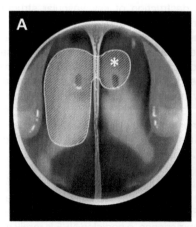
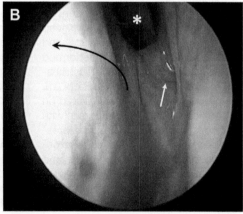

Fig. 1. Sinonasal examination before recurrent transsphenoidal surgery. (*A*) "1.5" approach to the sphenoid sinus with wide right-sided sphenoidotomy (*green shaded area*) and limited left-sided sphenoidotomy (*asterisk*) with preservation of inferiorly located nasal septal artery supply to the septum. (*B*) Left-sided sinonasal examination showing prior "1.5" approach with limited sphenoidotomy (*asterisk*) and preserved nasal septal artery branches (*white arrow*) to nasoseptal flap region (*curved black arrow*). (*Adapted from* Farrell CJ, Nyquist GG, Farag AA, et al. Principles of pituitary surgery. Otolaryngol Clin North Am. 2016;49(1):98; with permission.)

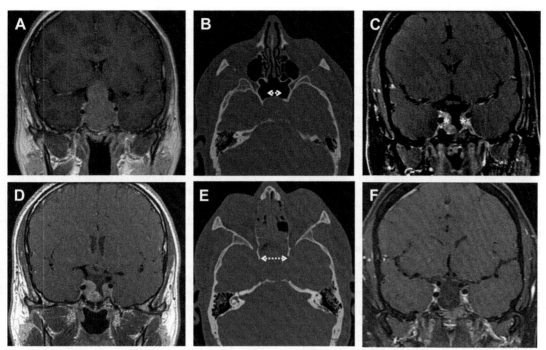

Fig. 2. Suboptimal surgical exposure. (*A*) Preoperative coronal MR image showing large pituitary macroadenoma without cavernous sinus invasion. (*B*) Postoperative CT scan showing inadequate anterior sella bony of removal (*arrow*) to access lateral aspects of adenoma. (*C*) Postoperative MR image showing residual adenoma (*asterisk*) along medial cavernous sinus walls bilaterally. (*D*) MR image showing delayed tumor progression. (*E*) Postoperative CT scan demonstrating wider bony removal (*arrow*) for revision surgery. (*F*) Postoperative MR image showing complete resection following revision surgery.

the carotid Doppler as well as frequent localization with neuronavigation to avoid vascular injury. Although we frequently remove the bone over the tuberculum sella, we do not typically proceed with opening of the dura over the planum sphenoidale and tuberculum sella until the intrasellar component of the tumor has been explored and the need for suprasellar transarachnoidal dissection deemed necessary to enable adequate tumor resection. An exception to the general approach is for patients with recurrent adenomas in the suprasellar region who have undergone prior transcranial resection. Schwartz[25] commented that once the outer rim of the adenoma consisting of the arachnoid, diaphragma sella, and pituitary gland have been transgressed during prior craniotomy, the residual or recurrent tumor becomes more adherent to surrounding structures such as the optic chiasm, optic nerves, and carotid artery branches. Anticipating these challenges, we routinely proceed with an extended transsphenoidal transtuberculum/transplanum approach to allow for early visualization of these structures and direct dissection. Residual tumor within the cavernous sinuses may be resected via either a medial or lateral cavernous sinus approach, a topic discussed more extensively in other articles

of this edition of *Neurosurgery Clinics*. It is important, however, to understand the long-term tumor control and complication rates associated with the various alternative therapies for recurrent pituitary adenomas, including radiation and medical therapies. As these alternative options continue to demonstrate increased efficacy and safety, it is becoming more difficult to justify the risks of cavernous sinus surgery for pituitary adenomas, especially for fibrous tumors. After tumor resection has been completed, the cavity should be inspected using direct visualization with angled endoscopes. If residual tumor is found, but not safely accessible, it may be necessary to expand the approach. In addition, if the diaphragma sella does not descend symmetrically, this may indicate that tumor resection is incomplete. After complete or maximally safe tumor resection has been confirmed, careful hemostasis is obtained. In our series of 61 endoscopic endonasal transsphenoidal surgeries for recurrent pituitary adenomas, 2 patients developed symptomatic postoperative hematomas with visual worsening requiring emergent surgical reintervention.[24] In our experience, the presence of residual tumor at the time of closure is the most significant factor influencing the likelihood of delayed bleeding complications.

In our series we also encountered an intraoperative CSF leak in 44% of patients, which is consistent with the more aggressive resections performed for these recurrent tumors and the often larger size of the tumors at the time of repeat surgical intervention. The postoperative CSF leak rate in this series was 4.9%, which is similar to the rates reported in other large contemporary revision endoscopic transsphenoidal series for pituitary adenomas.[21] Whether in a primary or revision setting, the main objective of sellar reconstruction after pituitary surgery is to minimize the risk of postoperative CSF leak and associated complications such as meningitis. As the risk of leak varies with a multitude of associated clinical factors, reconstructive strategies should be tailored to the individual patient. Within the armamentarium of the skull base surgeon exists a wide variety of reconstructive techniques and materials. These range from simple, single-layered techniques such as free mucosal grafts to more complex, multilayered closures involving vascularized tissue. Graft materials include a variety of both autologous (mucosa, nasal septum cartilage or bone, abdominal fat, and fascia lata) and synthetic (dural substitutes, bone cement, and dural sealants) options. When used appropriately, there is good evidence to suggest that these techniques may be effective.[13,33–35]

Reconstructive approaches should focus on identifying patients with a higher inherent risk of postoperative CSF leak who require more robust reconstructions. At the authors' institution, patients are stratified into low-risk, intermediate-risk, and high-risk groups.[24] The low-risk group consists of those cases without an apparent intraoperative CSF leak, in which case either an onlay of oxidized cellulose (Surgicel [Ethicon, Somerville, NJ, USA]) alone or an inlay collagen graft with epidural dural sealant is used depending on the size of the dural defect and degree of diaphragm descent after tumor resection. The intermediate-risk group consists of those with low-flow CSF leaks, which are generally repaired with an inlay collagen graft and epidural dural sealant. The high-risk group consists of those with large defects with wide opening of the suprasellar cistern or third ventricle, as encountered in expanded approaches, and are repaired with a fascia lata inlay/onlay "button graft" followed by a pedicle NSF, dural sealant, and absorbable packing.[36]

RADIATION THERAPY FOR RECURRENT PITUITARY ADENOMAS

Adjuvant radiation therapy is a crucial component in the treatment of residual and recurrent pituitary adenomas and is typically delivered using stereotactic radiosurgery (SRS), conventional conformal radiotherapy, or fractionated stereotactic radiotherapy (FSRT). The goals of radiation therapy are to achieve tumor control for NFPAs and tumor control with endocrine remission for functional adenomas. SRS is the most common modality used to treat recurrent pituitary adenomas and is typically delivered in a single session with a marginal dose of 12 to 18 Gy. Tumor control rates are reported as 94% to 100% at 5 years and 76% to 87% at 10 years of follow-up for NFPAs.[37] Postradiation neurologic deficits and hypopituitarism following SRS may develop in up to 7% and 39% of patients, respectively.[38] Although uncommon, additional potential complications of radiation therapy include symptomatic radiation necrosis, secondary neoplasms, and radiation-induced vasculopathy.[39]

Delayed-onset endocrinopathy has been associated with increased tumor volume and preradiation function of the pituitary gland. Cranial neuropathies, specifically optic nerve complications, have been associated with radiation doses to the optic chiasm of greater than 8 to 12 Gy, which may result from tumor proximity to the optic apparatus.[40,41] In general, a 3- to 5-mm margin is necessary between the optic apparatus and the recurrent tumor to safely perform single-session radiosurgery. When the adenoma is proximally associated with the optic chiasm or other dose-limiting radiosensitive structure such as the brainstem, radiation hypofractionation may be used to decrease radiation-induced toxicity. Fractionation permits the delivery of higher total doses of radiation separated over multiple smaller doses to minimize toxicity by a slower rate of delivery. FSRT is also frequently used for larger tumor volumes and tumors with highly irregular contours whereby maintenance of larger doses over a wider radiation field may be necessary to decrease the risk of recurrence.[42] Treatment outcomes of pituitary adenomas with FSRT have been favorable, resulting in excellent long-term control rates of greater than 95% at 5 years,[43–45] and a recent consensus statement by the Congress of Neurologic Surgeons emphasized the utility of adjuvant radiation therapy, either SRS or FSRT, in decreasing the rate of recurrence for NFPAs.[46] Although comparison studies of SRS and FSRT have supported the equivalent effectiveness in long-term tumor control, the rates of new endocrinopathy with FSRT have not been well established.

Because of the uncertain natural history of residual pituitary adenomas and the potential complications of radiation therapy, SRS and FSRT are frequently delayed for tumor remnants after subtotal surgical resection until there is evidence of radiographic or symptomatic progression. Delaying radiation treatment, however, may result in increased tumor volumes and consequent increased likelihood of radiation-related visual complications caused by abutment or compression of the optic apparatus and new endocrinopathy resulting from compression of the normal gland or higher radiation doses to the gland. Recently, 2 studies described experiences with early versus late SRS for treatment of recurrent or residual NFPAs.[47,48] In both studies, tumor control rates were excellent and rates of new endocrinopathy seemed to be lower when SRS was administered earlier as adjuvant therapy for residual tumors rather than as delayed therapy for recurrent progressive pituitary adenomas. Pomeraniec and colleagues[47] found a significantly increased likelihood of developing new endocrinopathy in the delayed cohort of up to 64%, which the investigators attributed to the effects from tumor progression. Similarly, Sadik and colleagues[48] performed a retrospective study comparing early adjuvant SRS (<6 months) for treatment of residual NFPAs following subtotal surgical resection with delayed SRS at the time of radiographic progression. Intratumoral bleeding and swelling occurred in 2% and 4% of the early and delayed SRS groups, respectively. Delayed treatment also resulted in a higher proportion of new endocrinopathy (18%) compared with early treatment (4%), with these findings potentially related to increased tumor volumes at the time of recurrence. Though it certainly remains reasonable to delay radiation therapy for residual and recurrent pituitary adenomas, early prescription of radiation treatment should be strongly considered for aggressive adenoma pathologic subtypes and for those tumors exhibiting faster than anticipated recurrences and growth rates.

Radiation therapy also plays an important role in inducing hormonal remission for recurrent functional adenomas resistant to medical therapies and not amenable to further surgery. Endocrine remission rates for corticotropin-secreting adenomas with SRS range from 28% to 70% with higher radiation doses necessary to induce remission compared with those necessary for tumor control with NFPAs.[37] A recently reported retrospective multicenter cohort study involving 278 patients demonstrated a 64% rate of durable hypercortisolism control at 10 years using a median margin dose of 23.7 Gy.[49] The mean time to cortisol normalization after SRS was 14.5 months. The reported remission rates for acromegaly range from 17% to 58% at 5 years, with differences in reported rates likely related to evolution in remission criteria over time. The time interval for endocrine remission after SRS is typically longer for acromegaly than for Cushing disease, with the same collaborative multicenter group reporting a mean time to durable endocrine remission of 38 months.[50]

MEDICAL THERAPY FOR TREATMENT-REFRACTORY RECURRENT PITUITARY ADENOMAS

Most pituitary tumors exhibit benign behavior and can be effectively controlled with surgery and radiation therapy. However, up to 35% of adenomas have invasive characteristics at the time of surgery with invasion of the surrounding dura, bone, sphenoid sinus, and cavernous sinuses.[51] Although the latest WHO classification system has provided new biomarkers of clinically aggressive behavior, predicting future tumor growth patterns and response to therapy remains uncertain. No single morphologic feature is available to predict pituitary carcinomas, and these fortunately rare tumors continue to be defined by their demonstration of metastatic spread.[11] Management of patients with these aggressive pituitary adenomas and pituitary carcinomas that prove refractory to standard therapies requires consultation with knowledgeable and experienced multidisciplinary teams.

To date, the most commonly used and effective medical therapy for refractory tumors is temozolomide (TMZ), an oral alkylating agent typically administered for the treatment of malignant gliomas. The 2018 European Society of Endocrinology (ESE) clinical guidelines recommend TMZ as first-line therapy for tumors based on a pooled review of 106 reported patients treated with TMZ with an overall volume reduction of 47%.[52] Complete tumor regression was observed in 5%, including 5 patients with pituitary carcinomas. The ESE recommends that TMZ be administered according to the standard dosing regimen of 150 to 200 mg/m^2 for 5 consecutive days every 28 days. Response to treatment on neuroimaging should be assessed after 3 dosing cycles and responders continued on TMZ for at least 6 months. Assessment of tumor DNA repair enzyme O^6-methylguanine methyltransferase (MGMT) expression by immunohistochemistry is recommended to predict response to TMZ, with high levels of MGMT correlated with decreased response.

Very few data are available to guide second-line treatment of TMZ-resistant pituitary tumors. The ESE recommends consideration of potential molecular targeted therapies toward the mTOR (mammalian target of rapamycin), EGFR (epidermal growth factor receptor), and VEGF (vascular endothelial growth factor) pathways. Dopamine agonist (DA) therapy may also be potentially effective for progressive NFPAs because of the expression of dopamine-2 receptor on these tumors.[53,54] Greenman and colleagues[53] reported among patients with progressive tumor following subtotal resection, 58% achieved tumor control with DA therapy. Among patients treated with DA as preventive therapy following subtotal resection, 87% maintained stable tumor size or shrinkage, which was significantly improved in comparison with the control group experience (47% tumor control).

A potential emerging therapy for standard treatment of refractory pituitary adenomas is the use of immunotherapy. A recent study by Wang and colleagues[55] reported that programmed death-ligand 1 (PD-L1), a key predictive marker of immunotherapy response, is frequently expressed in functional pituitary adenomas with higher Ki-67 index. PD-L1 expression was detected in 59% of functional tumors compared with 34% of NFPAs. Similarly, Mei and colleagues[56] showed significantly higher levels of PD-L1 expression and tumor-infiltrating lymphocytes in functional tumors, further raising the possibility that checkpoint blockade immunotherapy may be effective in cases of functional adenomas refractory to conventional management.

REFERENCES

1. Dekkers OM, Pereira AM, Romijn JA. Treatment and follow-up of clinically nonfunctioning pituitary macroadenomas. J Clin Endocrinol Metab 2008;93(10): 3717–26.

2. Vance ML. Treatment of patients with a pituitary adenoma: one clinician's experience. Neurosurg Focus 2004;16(4):E1.

3. Mattozo CA, Dusick JR, Esposito F, et al. Suboptimal sphenoid and sellar exposure: a consistent finding in patients treated with repeat transsphenoidal surgery for residual endocrine-inactive macroadenomas. Neurosurgery 2006;58(5):857–65 [discussion: 857–65].

4. Dickerman RD, Oldfield EH. Basis of persistent and recurrent Cushing disease: an analysis of findings at repeated pituitary surgery. J Neurosurg 2002;97(6): 1343–9.

5. Roelfsema F, Biermasz NR, Pereira AM. Clinical factors involved in the recurrence of pituitary adenomas after surgical remission: a structured review and meta-analysis. Pituitary 2012;15(1):71–83.

6. Cappabianca P, Solari D. The endoscopic endonasal approach for the treatment of recurrent or

7. Cavallo LM, Solari D, Tasiou A, et al. Endoscopic endonasal transsphenoidal removal of recurrent and regrowing pituitary adenomas: experience on a 59-patient series. World Neurosurg 2013;80(3–4): 342–50.

8. Chang EF, Zada G, Kim S, et al. Long-term recurrence and mortality after surgery and adjuvant radiotherapy for nonfunctional pituitary adenomas. J Neurosurg 2008;108(4):736–45.

9. Rosen MR, Saigal K, Evans J, et al. A review of the endoscopic approach to the pituitary through the sphenoid sinus. Curr Opin Otolaryngol Head Neck Surg 2006;14(1):6–13.

10. Lopes MBS. The 2017 World Health Organization classification of tumors of the pituitary gland: a summary. Acta Neuropathol 2017;134(4):521–35.

11. Mete O, Lopes MB. Overview of the 2017 WHO classification of pituitary tumors. Endocr Pathol 2017; 28(3):228–43.

12. Cappabianca P, Alfieri A, Colao A, et al. Endoscopic endonasal transsphenoidal surgery in recurrent and residual pituitary adenomas: technical note. Minim Invasive Neurosurg 2000;43(1):38–43.

13. Tabaee A, Anand VK, Barron Y, et al. Endoscopic pituitary surgery: a systematic review and meta-analysis. J Neurosurg 2009;111(3):545–54.

14. Barker FG 2nd, Klibanski A, Swearingen B. Transsphenoidal surgery for pituitary tumors in the United States, 1996-2000: mortality, morbidity, and the effects of hospital and surgeon volume. J Clin Endocrinol Metab 2003;88(10):4709–19.

15. Alahmadi H, Dehdashti AR, Gentili F. Endoscopic endonasal surgery in recurrent and residual pituitary adenomas after microscopic resection. World Neurosurg 2012;77(3–4):540–7.

16. Hwang JM, Kim YH, Kim JW, et al. Feasibility of endoscopic endonasal approach for recurrent pituitary adenomas after microscopic trans-sphenoidal approach. J Korean Neurosurg Soc 2013;54(4): 317–22.

17. Jahangiri A, Wagner J, Han SW, et al. Morbidity of repeat transsphenoidal surgery assessed in more than 1000 operations. J Neurosurg 2014;121(1): 67–74.

18. Rudnik A, Zawadzki T, Galuszka-Ignasiak B, et al. Endoscopic transsphenoidal treatment in recurrent and residual pituitary adenomas—first experience. Minim Invasive Neurosurg 2006;49(1):10–4.

19. Tajudeen BA, Mundi J, Suh JD, et al. Endoscopic endonasal surgery for recurrent pituitary tumors: technical challenges to the surgical approach. J Neurol Surg B Skull Base 2015;76(1):50–6.

20. Wilson TJ, McKean EL, Barkan AL, et al. Repeat endoscopic transsphenoidal surgery for

residual pituitary adenomas: widening what to see expands what to do? World Neurosurg 2012;77(3–4):455–6.

acromegaly: remission and complications. Pituitary 2013;16(4):459–64.

21. Heringer LC, de Oliveira MF, Rotta JM, et al. Effect of repeated transsphenoidal surgery in recurrent or residual pituitary adenomas: a systematic review and meta-analysis. Surg Neurol Int 2016;7:14.

22. Kuo JS, Barkhoudarian G, Farrell CJ, et al. Congress of neurological surgeons systematic review and evidence-based guideline on surgical techniques and technologies for the management of patients with nonfunctioning pituitary adenomas. Neurosurgery 2016;79(4):E536–8.

23. Esquenazi Y, Essayed WI, Singh H, et al. Endoscopic endonasal versus microscopic transsphenoidal surgery for recurrent and/or residual pituitary adenomas. World Neurosurg 2017;101:186–95.

24. Do H, Kshettry VR, Siu A, et al. Extent of resection, visual, and endocrinologic outcomes for endoscopic endonasal surgery for recurrent pituitary adenomas. World Neurosurg 2017;102:35–41.

25. Schwartz TH. A role for centers of excellence in transsphenoidal surgery. World Neurosurg 2013; 80(3–4):270–1.

26. Jahangiri A, Wagner JR, Pekmezci M, et al. A comprehensive long-term retrospective analysis of silent corticotrophic adenomas vs hormone-negative adenomas. Neurosurgery 2013;73(1):8–17 [discussion: 17–8].

27. Farrell CJ, Nyquist GG, Farag AA, et al. Principles of pituitary surgery. Otolaryngol Clin North Am 2016; 49(1):95–106.

28. Zanation AM, Carrau RL, Snyderman CH, et al. Nasoseptal flap takedown and reuse in revision endoscopic skull base reconstruction. Laryngoscope 2011;121(1):42–6.

29. Patel MR, Taylor RJ, Hackman TG, et al. Beyond the nasoseptal flap: outcomes and pearls with secondary flaps in endoscopic endonasal skull base reconstruction. Laryngoscope 2014;124(4): 846–52.

30. Zada G, Du R, Laws ER Jr. Defining the "edge of the envelope": patient selection in treating complex sellar-based neoplasms via transsphenoidal versus open craniotomy. J Neurosurg 2011; 114(2):286–300.

31. Garcia HG, Otten M, Pyfer M, et al. Minimizing septectomy for endoscopic transsphenoidal approaches to the sellar and suprasellar regions: a cadaveric morphometric study. J Neurol Surg B Skull Base 2016;77(6):479–84.

32. Oldfield EH, Vortmeyer AO. Development of a histological pseudocapsule and its use as a surgical capsule in the excision of pituitary tumors. J Neurosurg 2006;104(1):7–19.

33. Gagliardi F, Boari N, Mortini P. Reconstruction techniques in skull base surgery. J Craniofac Surg 2011; 22(3):1015–20.

34. Tabaee A, Anand VK, Brown SM, et al. Algorithm for reconstruction after endoscopic pituitary and skull base surgery. Laryngoscope 2007;117(7): 1133–7.

35. Kuan EC, Yoo F, Patel PB, et al. An algorithm for sellar reconstruction following the endoscopic endonasal approach: a review of 300 consecutive cases. J Neurol Surg B Skull Base 2018;79(2):177–83.

36. Luginbuhl AJ, Campbell PG, Evans J, et al. Endoscopic repair of high-flow cranial base defects using a bilayer button. Laryngoscope 2010;120(5): 876–80.

37. Lee CC, Sheehan JP. Advances in gamma knife radiosurgery for pituitary tumors. Curr Opin Endocrinol Diabetes Obes 2016;23(4):331–8.

38. Sheehan JP, Xu Z, Lobo MJ. External beam radiation therapy and stereotactic radiosurgery for pituitary adenomas. Neurosurg Clin N Am 2012;23(4): 571–86.

39. Delgado-Lopez PD, Pi-Barrio J, Duenas-Polo MT, et al. Recurrent non-functioning pituitary adenomas: a review on the new pathological classification, management guidelines and treatment options. Clin Transl Oncol 2018;20(10):1233–45.

40. Sheehan JP, Niranjan A, Sheehan JM, et al. Stereotactic radiosurgery for pituitary adenomas: an intermediate review of its safety, efficacy, and role in the neurosurgical treatment armamentarium. J Neurosurg 2005;102(4):678–91.

41. Mayo C, Martel MK, Marks LB, et al. Radiation dose-volume effects of optic nerves and chiasm. Int J Radiat Oncol Biol Phys 2010;76(3 Suppl): S28–35.

42. Losa M, Bogazzi F, Cannavo S, et al. Temozolomide therapy in patients with aggressive pituitary adenomas or carcinomas. J Neurooncol 2016;126(3): 519–25.

43. Scheick S, Amdur RJ, Kirwan JM, et al. Long-term outcome after fractionated radiotherapy for pituitary adenoma: the curse of the secretory tumor. Am J Clin Oncol 2016;39(1):49–54.

44. Minniti G, Scaringi C, Poggi M, et al. Fractionated stereotactic radiotherapy for large and invasive non-functioning pituitary adenomas: long-term clinical outcomes and volumetric MRI assessment of tumor response. Eur J Endocrinol 2015;172(4): 433–41.

45. Iwata H, Sato K, Tatewaki K, et al. Hypofractionated stereotactic radiotherapy with CyberKnife for nonfunctioning pituitary adenoma: high local control with low toxicity. Neuro Oncol 2011;13(8):916–22.

46. Sheehan J, Lee CC, Bodach ME, et al. Congress of neurological surgeons systematic review and evidence-based guideline for the management of patients with residual or recurrent nonfunctioning pituitary adenomas. Neurosurgery 2016;79(4): E539–40.

47. Pomeraniec IJ, Dallapiazza RF, Xu Z, et al. Early versus late Gamma Knife radiosurgery following transsphenoidal resection for nonfunctioning pituitary macroadenomas: a matched cohort study. J Neurosurg 2016;125(1):202–12.

48. Sadik ZHA, Voormolen EHJ, Depauw P, et al. Treatment of nonfunctional pituitary adenoma postoperative remnants: adjuvant or delayed gamma knife radiosurgery? World Neurosurg 2017;100:361–8.

49. Mehta GU, Ding D, Patibandla MR, et al. Stereotactic radiosurgery for cushing disease: results of an international, multicenter study. J Clin Endocrinol Metab 2017;102(11):4284–91.

50. Ding D, Mehta GU, Patibandla MR, et al. Stereotactic radiosurgery for acromegaly: an international multicenter retrospective cohort study. Neurosurgery 2019;84(3):717–25.

51. Hansen TM, Batra S, Lim M, et al. Invasive adenoma and pituitary carcinoma: a SEER database analysis. Neurosurg Rev 2014;37(2):279–85 [discussion: 285–6].

52. McCormack A, Dekkers OM, Petersenn S, et al. Treatment of aggressive pituitary tumours and carcinomas: results of a European Society of Endocrinology (ESE) survey 2016. Eur J Endocrinol 2018; 178(3):265–76.

53. Greenman Y, Cooper O, Yaish I, et al. Treatment of clinically nonfunctioning pituitary adenomas with dopamine agonists. Eur J Endocrinol 2016;175(1): 63–72.

54. Gabalec F, Beranek M, Netuka D, et al. Dopamine 2 receptor expression in various pathological types of clinically non-functioning pituitary adenomas. Pituitary 2012;15(2):222–6.

55. Wang PF, Wang TJ, Yang YK, et al. The expression profile of PD-L1 and CD8(+) lymphocyte in pituitary adenomas indicating for immunotherapy. J Neurooncol 2018;139(1):89–95.

56. Mei Y, Bi WL, Greenwald NF, et al. Increased expression of programmed death ligand 1 (PD-L1) in human pituitary tumors. Oncotarget 2016;7(47): 76565–76.

Visual Outcomes After Pituitary Surgery

Benjamin Uy, MD, PhD, Bayard Wilson, MD, Wi Jin Kim, MD, Giyarpuram Prashant, MD, Marvin Bergsneider, MD*

KEYWORDS

- Postoperative visual recovery • Visual outcomes • Visual acuity • Visual field
- Endoscopic endonasal surgery • Factors for recovery

KEY POINTS

- Following endoscopic endonasal pituitary surgery, most patients have improvement in visual symptoms such as visual fields or visual acuity.
- Most visual field recovery occurs within the first 3 to 6 months.
- Preoperative factors such as retinal nerve fiber layer thickness, severity of the preoperative deficit, duration of visual symptoms, tumor size, extent of resection, and patient age may serve as predictors of postoperative visual outcomes.
- Intraoperative considerations and techniques are important to optimize visual outcomes for safe decompression of the optic chiasm and nerve.

VISUAL MANIFESTATIONS OF PITUITARY TUMORS

Clinical manifestations of pituitary tumors generally fall into 1 of 2 categories: (1) signs and symptoms related to pituitary gland dysfunction, such as underproduction or overproduction of hormones produced and/or secreted by the pituitary gland, and (2) signs and symptoms related to mechanical effects of tumor expansion beyond the sella turcica.[1] Visual signs and symptoms are almost exclusively the result of the latter category. The incidence of visual symptoms among patients with pituitary tumors has been reported to vary widely,[2] although a recent study found that approximately 41% of pituitary tumor patients first present to a physician with complaints primarily related to vision.[3]

The classic visual disturbance associated with pituitary tumors is a bitemporal hemianopsia (**Fig. 1**), in which bilateral temporal visual fields are affected. This pattern occurs when the body of the chiasm (consisting of the crossing nasal fibers of each optic nerve) is severely compressed by a superiorly extending tumor.[3] It has been theorized that bitemporal field defects caused by pituitary tumors, specifically those found in patients with preserved acuity and color perception, result from ischemia to the optic chiasm rather than direct compression, given that the lateral and middle portions of the optic chiasm are known to have separate arterial blood supplies.[4,5] This defect can be complete (ie, involving the entire hemifield) or partial, typically starting with the superior hemifield (ie, superior temporal quadrantinopsia) and progressing inferiorly (**Fig. 2**). Several different visual field deficit patterns have been reported,[6,7] and all relate to the position of the growing tumor relative to the optic nerves and chiasm.[3] Unilateral field defects are not uncommon, and these patients are more likely to have nasal field defects than patients with bilateral pathology.[3] Mixed

Disclosure Statement: The authors have nothing to disclose.
Department of Neurosurgery, University California Los Angeles, 300 Stein Plaza Driveway #420, Los Angeles, CA 90095, USA
* Corresponding author.
E-mail address: mbergsneider@mednet.ucla.edu

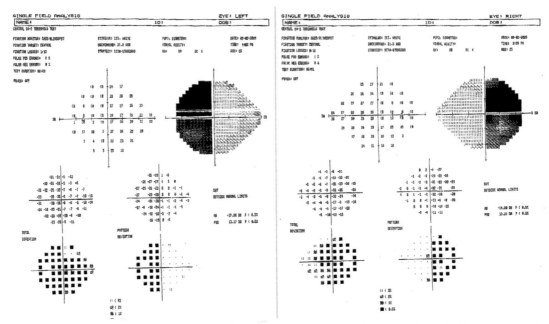

Fig. 1. Humphrey visual fields in a patient with a large pituitary macroadenoma with optic chiasm compression displays bitemporal hemianopsia, with loss of vision in the bilateral temporal fields.

patterns of visual loss (ie, a central scotoma in one eye with a contralateral temporal or superotemporal field defect) have also been reported.[3] Ultimately, the pattern of visual field loss largely reflects the location of the chiasm in relation to the expanding tumor. Tumors compressing the optic tract posterior to the chiasm are more likely to present with homonymous defects, while those with compression anterior to the chiasm can result in mixed or unilateral visual field defects. Therefore, the anatomic orientation of the optic chiasm in relation to the sella plays a role in the resulting

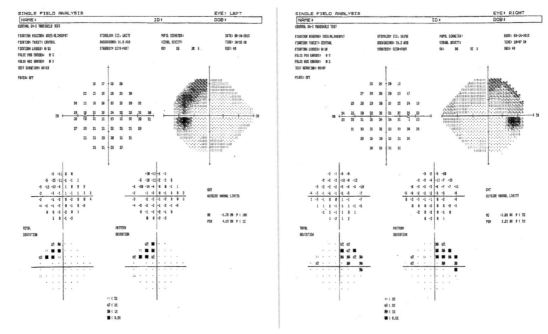

Fig. 2. Preoperative visual field testing revealed a loss of vision primarily in the bilateral superior temporal fields.

visual symptoms. Unilateral defects tend to be the least common, reports in the literature range from 1% to 13% of patients with visual field defects from pituitary tumors.[3]

In addition to disturbances in visual fields, pituitary tumors are known to present with changes in visual acuity or color vision. Patients with visual field defects may report a decrease in visual acuity but have normal or near-normal acuity on formal examination.[3] Central scotomas and color vision disturbances are typically less common than visual field disturbances, which can be explained by the fact that nerve fibers subserving central vision (ie, the macula) run more centrally within the optic nerve and chiasm than those subserving peripheral vision, and as such manifest compressive symptoms generally after peripheral vision fibers have already been affected.[6] Peripheral visual field testing therefore is the most sensitive ophthalmologic test for detecting optic pathway compromise secondary to a pituitary tumor.[6] That said, measurable decreases in visual acuity or color perception do occur, and have been reported in anywhere from 42% to 88% and 35% to 71% of patients with visual complaints, respectively.[8] In routine formal color vision testing, ophthalmologists will examine a small portion of the central visual field; in this small area, damage to the receptor layer from optic nerve compression tends to produce diminished red sensitivity (specifically a type 2 red-green defect).[5]

Fundoscopic examination is an important component of the physical assessment of patients with pituitary tumors, as it can reveal optic atrophy or papilledema. Optic atrophy, visible on examination as pallor of the optic disc, is more common, and occurs in cases of long-term compression of the optic nerve. Papilledema is exceedingly rare, as intracranial pressure elevation occurs in those sporadic cases of tumor extension so significant as to affect ventricular cerebrospinal fluid (CSF) outflow.[5,9,10] Pupillary examination is similarly important, as a poor response to light with normal constriction on accommodation can occur in cases of significant visual impairment. A more sensitive test for detecting early optic nerve damage is to elucidate a relative afferent pupillary defect (APD), although this test is only positive in cases of unilateral or asymmetric involvement of the optic tracts, and thus often correlates to asymmetric disturbances in visual field fields and/or acuity.[9]

Optical coherence tomography (OCT) is an important noninvasive tool to measure the thickness of retinal nerve fiber layer (RNFL) around the optic nerve head. RNFL thickness can serve as a preoperative prognostic marker for visual field recovery and means of tracking postoperative recovery. Many but not all patients with visual field deficits exhibit thinning of RNFL.[11] Patients with visual field deficits and normal preoperative RNFL thickness demonstrated greater and earlier VF improvement compared with thin RNFL.[12–15] Patients with improved visual fields also tended to show increased RNFL thickness postoperatively.

Finally, in rare cases, patients with pituitary tumors may present with ocular palsies or a depression of the corneal reflex, both of which can occur in cases of lateral tumor expansion to involve the cavernous sinus or trigeminal nerve, respectively.[6,9] These findings are exceedingly rare in cases of pituitary adenomas, with the exception of pituitary apoplexy.[9]

Given this range of visual manifestations, the authors concur with the recommendations put forth by consensus guidelines of a national neurosurgery organization that all patients undergo a thorough ophthalmologic evaluation prior to proceeding with surgical resection of a pituitary tumor.[16] This includes pupillary examination, extraocular movements, visual acuity and color vision, visual fields, and fundoscopic examination. This allows for detection of subtle neurologic deficits of which patients may not be consciously aware and serves as a baseline study to track visual improvements or deterioration over time.

INTRAOPERATIVE CONSIDERATIONS

Although there have not been major studies evaluating intraoperative technical considerations and visual outcomes after pituitary surgery, there are several aspects of pituitary surgery that are key to optimizing visual outcomes. As discussed previously, baseline visual deficits must be investigated thoroughly through an ophthalmologic examination. It is important to review all preoperative imaging to determine lateral and superior extent of tumor and contact with the optic apparatus. In addition, tumor involvement of the optic canal is a key consideration, particularly in the management of macroadenomas. This detailed review of imaging serves to guide a discussion with the patient regarding the primary goals of the surgery, whether it be gross total resection or decompression of the optic apparatus.

During surgical exposure, it is important to identify key landmarks early, including the medial and lateral opticocarotid recesses and inferior aspect of the optic canal bony covering over the optic nerves. This is a key step in guiding bony exposure and preservation of the optic nerves. When removing the bone covering the sellar face, it is important not to significantly push the sellar dura if there is a preoperative visual field deficit. Doing so, typically with Kerrison rongeurs, may indirectly impinge the optic chiasm by elevating the tumor mass.

For most pituitary tumors with suprasellar extension, the diaphragma sella is intact. A smooth dome-like appearance of the suprasellar component (**Fig. 3**) indicates that the suprasellar extension is contained beneath the diaphragma sella. With careful dissection and removal of the tumor, the diaphragma remains intact and prolapses into the sellar cavity. As the diaphragma is not attached or adherent to the optic apparatus, the optic chiasm and nerves are decompressed without the need to directly manipulate these structures. If only part of the diaphragma descends, care must be taken when exploring the retained tumor to not compress the optic structures.

Invasive tumors with supradiaphragmatic extension deserve special attention. This component of the tumor mass may be in the pre- or subchiasmatic cistern, directly touching the optic nerves or chiasm (**Fig. 4**). Microsurgical principles of dissection should be used to free the tumor

capsule, in order to preserve the arachnoid and pial blood supply to the chiasm (**Fig. 5**). There are often multiple superior hypophyseal vessels that perfuse the optic apparatus in this region, in addition to feeders from the anterior cerebral artery and posterior communicating artery, and these should all be preserved. After tumor removal, a thorough inspection of the cavity ensures hemostasis and decompression of the optic chiasm.

In rare cases, removal of tumors with large suprasellar extension projecting posteriorly can result in prolapse of the optic chiasm into the sellar space, manifesting with postoperative blindness.[17]

VISUAL OUTCOMES AFTER PITUITARY SURGERY

Following resection of pituitary adenomas in patients with baseline visual field deficits, visual fields appear to recover in 3 stages: rapid recovery (minutes to days), delayed recovery (weeks to months), and late recovery (months to years). Rapid recovery is attributed to alleviation of conduction blockade, while delayed/late recovery is due to remyelination and restoration of axon transportation, resulting in recovery of the retinal ganglion cells.[18] Resection of tumors has been associated with increased visual-related quality of life in a series of patients on 1 study.[19]

Multiple studies have shown visual field improvements varying from 79% to 95% postoperatively after endoscopic endonasal resection of pituitary adenomas, with a recent meta-analysis in 2017 showing 80.8% improvement.[12,20–22] Improvement ranges from complete resolution and normalization to mild improvement in visual field deficit. Recovery is variable, and 1 study showed improvement as far as 5 years after surgery; most improvement, however, occurs within the first 3 to 6 months.[23] Visual acuity has also reported to improve in 45% to 86% of cases, with 1 meta-analysis reporting improvement in 67.5% of cases.

Upper temporal fields are most affected by pituitary adenomas because of the upward compression of pituitary tumors on the optic chiasm, followed by the lower temporal and nasal fields.[23] Similarly, recovery follows a similar pattern. Tumors typically greater than 2 cm in diameter present with visual symptoms, and some studies have referenced an associated 8 to 10 mm in the sagittal plane above the frontal base and posterior clinoid process and 12 to 13 mm in the coronal plane above the upper surface of the bilateral internal carotid artery.[21,24,25] Large adenomas and

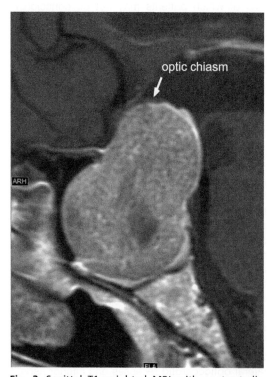

Fig. 3. Sagittal T1-weighted MRI with contrast displays a large pituitary macroadenoma with a sellar and suprasellar component. The smooth dome-like appearance of the suprasellar component suggests that the suprasellar extension is contained beneath the diaphragma sella. Note the optic chiasm draped over the anterosuperior portion of the tumor.

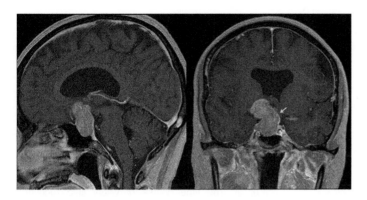

Fig. 4. Sagittal and coronal T1-weighted postcontrast MRI displays a pituitary macroadenoma with significant suprasellar component. The optic chiasm is elevated superiorly and compressed to the left. The optic chiasm is elevated superiorly and compressed to the left (*white arrow*).

giant adenoma resection are associated with improvement of visual symptoms; however, these tumors still result in worse visual outcomes compared with smaller adenomas.[24]

Preoperative factors such as severity of visual defects, duration of visual symptoms, tumor size, extent of resection, patient age, surgeon experience, and RNFL thickness have been suspected to be predictive of postoperative vision change.[12,20,26–28] Focusing on operative approach, extent of resection was significant in 1 study during bivariate analysis of gross total resection versus subtotal resection.[29] In contrast, 1 study showed that patients with a greater extent of resection (89.9%) had worse visual acuity, while those with a smaller extent of resection (71.5%) had unchanged visual acuities. An average 83.4% resection was found in those who had visual acuity improvement.[30] In multiple other studies, the extent of resection was not significant for differences in visual outcomes.[23,27,31–33] Shorter duration and less severe preoperative

visual symptoms were found to be important factors that may be predictive for postoperative visual recovery.[23,26,34–38]

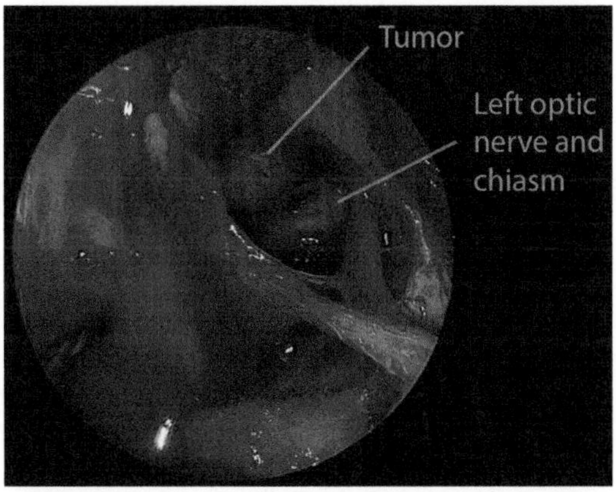

Of note, non-functioning pituitary adenomas have lower remission rates after surgery compared with functional tumors, likely because of the greater size at initial detection.[39] Nonfunctioning pituitary adenomas have a 10-year recurrence/persistence rate of around 16%, with approximately 6% requiring reoperation.[40] Although vertical suprasellar tumor size plays a greater role on visual field deficit, horizonal growth may be affiliated with recurrence, which has been attributed to difficulty of complete resection due to tumor extension toward the cavernous sinus.[24]

SUMMARY

Visual signs and symptoms are a common manifestation of pituitary adenomas. Although bitemporal hemlanopsla Is a classic presenting visual field deficit, there are several different visual disturbances that can result from these tumors. A thorough ophthalmologic evaluation should be performed in all patients prior to undergoing surgery. After pituitary surgery, most patients do have improvement in visual symptoms, with factors, including severity of preoperative deficit, duration of visual symptoms, tumor size, extent of resection, and patient age serving as predictors of postoperative visual outcomes.

REFERENCES

1. Arafah BM, Nasrallah MP. Pituitary tumors: pathophysiology, clinical manifestations and management. Endocr Relat Cancer 2001;8(4):287–305.
2. Bynke H. Pituitary adenomas with ocular manifestations AU - Bynke, Hans. Neuroophthalmol 1986;6(5): 303–11.
3. Ogra S, Nichols AD, Stylli S, et al. Visual acuity and pattern of visual field loss at presentation in pituitary adenoma. J Clin Neurosci 2014;21(5):735–40.

Fig. 5. Endoscopic intraoperative view of a sellar tumor extending to the chiasmatic cistern. The left optic nerve and chiasm are visible; note the pial vessels visible on the surface of the nerve.

Tumor

Left optic nerve and chiasm

4. Bergland R. The arterial supply of the human optic chiasm. J Neurosurg 1969;31(3):327–34.

5. Cruysberg JRM, Pinckers A. Acquired color vision defects in compressive optic neuropathy. Neuroophthalmol 1982;2(3):169–81.

6. Poon A, McNeill P, Harper A, et al. Patterns of visual loss associated with pituitary macroadenomas. Aust N Z J Ophthalmol 1995;23(2):107–15.

7. Wang H, Sun W, Fu Z, et al. The pattern of visual impairment in patients with pituitary adenoma. J Int Med Res 2008;36(5):1064–9.

8. Herse P. Pituitary macroadenoma: a case report and review. Clin Exp Optom 2014;97(2):125–32.

9. Powell M, Lightman SL, Laws ER. Management of pituitary tumors : the clinician's practical guide. 2nd edition. Totowa (NJ): Humana Press; 2003. xvi, 318.

10. Powell M. Recovery of vision following transsphenoidal surgery for pituitary adenomas. Br J Neurosurg 1995;9(3):367–73.

11. Johansson C, Lindblom B. The role of optical coherence tomography in the detection of pituitary adenoma. Acta Ophthalmol 2009;87(7):776–9.

12. Danesh-Meyer HV, Wong A, Papchenko T, et al. Optical coherence tomography predicts visual outcome for pituitary tumors. J Clin Neurosci 2015; 22(7):1098–104.

13. Zhang J, Zhang S, Song Y, et al. Predictive value of preoperative retinal nerve fiber layer thickness for postoperative visual recovery in patients with chiasmal compression. Oncotarget 2017;8(35): 59148–55.

14. Jacob M, Raverot G, Jouanneau E, et al. Predicting visual outcome after treatment of pituitary adenomas with optical coherence tomography. Am J Ophthalmol 2009;147(1):64–70.e2.

15. Garcia T, Sanchez S, Litré CF, et al. Prognostic value of retinal nerve fiber layer thickness for postoperative peripheral visual field recovery in optic chiasm compression. J Neurosurg 2014;121(1):165–9.

16. Newman SA, Turbin RE, Bodach ME, et al. Congress of neurological surgeons systematic review and evidence-based guideline on pretreatment ophthalmology evaluation in patients with suspected nonfunctioning pituitary adenomas. Neurosurgery 2016;79(4):E530–2.

17. Barrow DL, Tindall GT. Loss of vision after transsphenoidal surgery. Neurosurgery 1990;27(1):60–8.

18. Kerrison JB, Lynn MJ, Baer CA, et al. Stages of improvement in visual fields after pituitary tumor resection. Am J Ophthalmol 2000;130(6):813–20.

19. Okamoto Y, Okamoto F, Yamada S, et al. Vision-related quality of life after transsphenoidal surgery for pituitary adenoma. Invest Ophthalmol Vis Sci 2010;51(7):3405–10.

20. Sun M, Zhang ZQ, Ma CY, et al. Predictive factors of visual function recovery after pituitary adenoma resection: a literature review and meta-analysis. Int J Ophthalmol 2017;10(11):1742–50.

21. Monteiro ML, Zambon BK, Cunha LP. Predictive factors for the development of visual loss in patients with pituitary macroadenomas and for visual recovery after optic pathway decompression. Can J Ophthalmol 2010;45(4):404–8.

22. Jahangiri A, Lamborn KR, Blevins L, et al. Factors associated with delay to pituitary adenoma diagnosis in patients with visual loss. J Neurosurg 2012;116(2):283.

23. Gnanalingham KK, Bhattacharjee S, Pennington R, et al. The time course of visual field recovery following transsphenoidal surgery for pituitary adenomas: predictive factors for a good outcome. J Neurol Neurosurg Psychiatry 2005;76(3):415–9.

24. Ho RW, Huang HM, Ho JT. The influence of pituitary adenoma size on vision and visual outcomes after trans-sphenoidal adenectomy: a report of 78 cases. J Korean Neurosurg Soc 2015;57(1):23–31.

25. Ikeda H, Yoshimoto T. Visual disturbances in patients with pituitary adenoma. Acta Neurol Scand 1995;92(2):157–60.

26. Lee S, Kim SJ, Yu YS, et al. Prognostic factors for visual recovery after transsphenoidal pituitary adenectomy. Br J Neurosurg 2013;27(4):425–9.

27. Muskens IS, Zamanipoor Najafabadi AH, Briceno V, et al. Visual outcomes after endoscopic endonasal pituitary adenoma resection: a systematic review and meta-analysis. Pituitary 2017;20(5):539–52.

28. Moon CH, Hwang SC, Kim BT, et al. Visual prognostic value of optical coherence tomography and photopic negative response in chiasmal compression. Invest Ophthalmol Vis Sci 2011;52(11): 8527–33.

29. Fredes F, Undurraga G, Rojas P, et al. Visual outcomes after endoscopic pituitary surgery in patients presenting with preoperative visual deficits. J Neurol Surg B Skull Base 2017;78(6):461–5.

30. Juraschka K, Khan OH, Godoy BL, et al. Endoscopic endonasal transsphenoidal approach to large and giant pituitary adenomas: institutional experience and predictors of extent of resection. J Neurosurg 2014;121(1):75–83.

31. Chabot JD, Chakraborty S, Imbarrato G, et al. Evaluation of outcomes after endoscopic endonasal surgery for large and giant pituitary macroadenoma: a retrospective review of 39 consecutive patients. World Neurosurg 2015;84(4):978–88.

32. Marenco HA, Zymberg ST, Santos Rde P, et al. Surgical treatment of non-functioning pituitary macroadenomas by the endoscopic endonasal approach in the elderly. Arq Neuropsiquiatr 2015;73(9):764–9.

33. Nakao N, Itakura T. Surgical outcome of the endoscopic endonasal approach for non-functioning giant pituitary adenoma. J Clin Neurosci 2011;18(1): 71–5.

34. Anik I, Anik Y, Cabuk B, et al. Visual outcome of an endoscopic endonasal transsphenoidal approach in pituitary macroadenomas: quantitative assessment with diffusion tensor imaging early and long-term results. World Neurosurg 2018;112: e691–701.

35. Anik I, Anik Y, Koc K, et al. Evaluation of early visual recovery in pituitary macroadenomas after endoscopic endonasal transphenoidal surgery: quantitative assessment with diffusion tensor imaging (DTI). Acta Neurochir (Wien) 2011;153(4):831–42.

36. Cohen AR, Cooper PR, Kupersmith MJ, et al. Visual recovery after transsphenoidal removal of pituitary adenomas. Neurosurgery 1985;17(3):446–52.

37. Lee J, Kim SW, Kim DW, et al. Predictive model for recovery of visual field after surgery of pituitary adenoma. J Neurooncol 2016;130(1):155–64.

38. Luomaranta T, Raappana A, Saarela V, et al. Factors affecting the visual outcome of pituitary adenoma patients treated with endoscopic transsphenoidal surgery. World Neurosurg 2017;105:422–31.

39. Roelfsema F, Biermasz NR, Pereira AM. Clinical factors involved in the recurrence of pituitary adenomas after surgical remission: a structured review and meta-analysis. Pituitary 2012;15(1):71–83.

40. Jane JA Jr, Laws ER Jr. The surgical management of pituitary adenomas in a series of 3,093 patients. J Am Coll Surg 2001;193(6):651–9.

Endocrine Outcomes After Pituitary Surgery

Anshu Buttan, MD[a], Adam N. Mamelak, MD[b],*

KEYWORDS

- Pituitary surgery • Adrenal insufficiency • Growth hormone • Hypogonadism • Prolactin

KEY POINTS

- Hormonal deficiencies, if present, before surgery are unlikely to completely normalize after surgery. Hormonal deficiencies associated with hypersecretory states generally have greater chance of recovery of function.
- Perioperative steroids are generally not indicated in the absence of preoperative adrenal dysfunction and may actually worsen outcomes.
- Immediate postoperative hormonal evaluation can sometimes provide reassurance of cure. However, longitudinal follow-up and assessment of each hormonal axis are critical.
- When some hypersecretory tumors are treated (eg, Cushing disease and acromegaly), subsequent deficiency in these hormones may require replacement after surgery.

INTRODUCTION

Removal of tumors in the sellar and parasellar region is a well-established and highly successful surgical method. Although surgical removal via either the transsphenoidal or the transcranial route can often result in excellent surgical outcomes, several morbidities are commonly associated with these surgeries. The most frequent complications seen are those related to temporary or permanent abnormalities in the hypothalamic-pituitary axis (HPA) and related downstream hormones. This article outlines the major disorders of regulation seen after pituitary surgery and provides an overview of basic treatment strategies aimed to correct these abnormalities.

PREOPERATIVE ASSESSMENT AS AN INDICATOR OF POSTOPERATIVE FUNCTION

Hormonal deficits that are present before surgery are unlikely to be corrected by even the most successful surgical removal of tumor. Several studies indicate a 5% to 40% chance of normalization of any single hormone axis that was absent before surgery; slight improvement may be seen in about 49% cases.[1–3] In contrast, for hypersecretory tumors, the possibility of hormonal normalization is far more frequent, especially in patients without cavernous sinus invasion.[1,2,4]

POSTOPERATIVE ISSUES

Adrenal Axis

Role of perioperative steroids

There are a variety of ways to manage steroids perioperatively, ranging from empiric treatment with stress dose steroids with gradual taper to a complete steroid-sparing protocol.[5] The authors generally favor a steroid-sparing approach, in which steroids are not administered in the perioperative period in patients who have no evidence of preoperative adrenal insufficiency (AI) with an otherwise routine and uncomplicated surgery.[6]

In most patients with an intact HPA cortisol axis before surgery, postoperative cortisol levels are

Disclosure Statement: The authors have nothing to disclose.
[a] Department of Medicine, Division of Endocrinology, Cedars-Sinai Medical Center, 8700 Beverly Boulevard, Becker B-131, Los Angeles, CA 90048, USA; [b] Department of Neurosurgery, Cedars-Sinai Medical Center, 127 S San Vicente Boulevard, A6600, Los Angeles, CA 90048, USA
* Corresponding author.
E-mail address: Adam.Mamelak@cshs.org

normal or elevated, demonstrating an appropriate physiologic response to the stress of surgery.[7,8] There does not appear to be an increased incidence of postoperative AI or diabetes insipidus in patients who receive no perioperative steroid supplementation.[8,9] Moreover, there is an increased risk of osteopenia, bone derangement, morbidity, and potentially increased mortality with empiric perioperative steroids.[10,11] For these reasons, in the absence of suspected surgery-related pituitary gland or stalk damage, the authors do not recommend the use of perioperative steroid supplementation in patients with intact preoperative HPA axis.

Postoperative adrenal insufficiency

Preoperative AI is reported in 10% to 27% of sellar masses and is even more pronounced in aggressive pathologic conditions such as craniopharyngioma, with up to 58% of patients having secondary AI before surgery.[2,12,13] Recovery of adrenal function after surgery, however, is reported in only 15% to 20% of patients and is associated with younger age, smaller tumor size (<2 cm), nonfunctional tumors, normal blood pressure, and lack of intraoperative cerebrospinal fluid leak.[1,14] When adrenal function is intact preoperatively, development of postoperative secondary AI is reported in 4% to 9% of patients, and up to 18% may experience early transient AI.[1,15] The risk of developing AI likely also reflects tumor size, extension into surrounding structures, and aggressiveness of tumor as well as experience of the surgeon. Early postoperative hyponatremia may also be an indicator of inadequate endogenous cortisol and should raise the suspicion of underlying secondary AI.[16]

Evaluation of postoperative adrenal function

In cases whereby a steroid-sparing protocol is used, basal morning cortisol may be used to assess adrenal function in the early postoperative period. Data suggest that those with intact HPA axis before surgery return to baseline cortisol secretion 48 hours after surgery.[17] However, a basal morning cortisol is not diagnostic of AI, nor is there an agreed on parameter at which point glucocorticoids should be administered. Several studies have suggested a serum cortisol level cutoff of 4 μg/dL to initiate glucocorticoids, whereas a level of 10 to 15 μg/dL may indicate a relatively low risk of AI.[6,18] The use of the cosyntropin stimulation test in the early postoperative setting has not been validated and is not recommended.[19,20] A normal cosyntropin stimulation test in this setting reflects a functional adrenal gland, but does not confer additional information regarding hypothalamic or pituitary function.

In patients who are treated with perioperative steroids and tapered to maintenance dosing, formal dynamic testing is often performed several weeks after surgery. An alternative approach for those without preoperative AI would be a rapid taper off steroids in 2 to 3 days and reassessment of adrenal function on day 3 to 5 with a morning basal cortisol.[19]

At the authors' institution, patients with an unremarkable operative course and intact preoperative adrenal function are assessed 6 weeks after pituitary surgery, either with basal morning cortisol or more commonly with formal dynamic testing using a 250-μg cosyntropin stimulation test. The authors use a cutoff of serum cortisol greater than 18 μg/dL 30 minutes after administration to effectively rule out AI.

Postoperative treatment

If AI is suspected from clinical or biochemical evaluation, the authors typically initiate hydrocortisone 15 mg in the morning and 5 mg in the afternoon, although weight-based nomograms may also be used. Patients are continued on this dose until formal dynamic testing is done several weeks later as an outpatient to determine need for continued treatment. For persistent AI, hydrocortisone is then adjusted to optimize clinical need and minimize effects of supraphysiologic replacement. Long-term doses of 10 mg in the morning and 5 mg in the afternoon are most common but are adjusted to match patient-specific needs.

Cushing disease

Cushing disease (CD) is characterized as cortisol excess due to an ACTH-secreting pituitary adenomas. If surgery is curative, AI can be expected in the immediate (<7 day) postoperative period. Assessment of adrenal function in the early postoperative period is critical and should be assessed with either morning basal cortisol or 24-hour urine free cortisol within the first week of surgery.[21–23] In most instances, postoperative steroids are withheld to assess morning cortisol levels while the patient is still hospitalized. An alternate strategy is to initiate postoperative steroids with assessment of adrenal function 1 week after surgery in an ambulatory setting.[5]

Postoperative treatment of Cushing disease

Patients in remission should be started on steroids for AI. For those not in remission, repeat surgery is considered first-line therapy.[22,24,25] At the authors' institution, cortisol is assessed every 6 hours after surgery, and glucocorticoids are initiated if cortisol drops to less than 4 μg/dL. If tumor excision is not feasible, other options may include hemiphysectomy or total hypophysectomy, radiation, medical therapy, or bilateral adrenalectomy.

Thyroid Axis

When thyroid function is intact before surgery, the incidence of new postoperative hypothyroidism is approximately 3% and is often associated with other pituitary hormonal deficiencies.[1,3] However, only 7% of those with preexisting secondary hypothyroidism recover after surgery for nonfunctional tumors.[1] Secondary hypothyroidism is usually mild, because a small portion of thyroid gland function is independent of thyroid-stimulating hormone (TSH).[26]

Postoperative evaluation of thyroid function

If early postoperative thyroid dysfunction is suspected, both free thyroxine (FT4) or free thyroxine index and TSH should be obtained for evaluation. In secondary (or tertiary) hypothyroidism, TSH may be low or inappropriately normal in the setting of low peripheral thyroxine level, reflecting an inadequate response.[27] In the immediate postoperative period, early hyponatremia may be an indicator of thyroid dysfunction, although hyponatremia is often mild.[28,29] An important consideration is the administration of perioperative stress dose steroids or dopamine agonist therapy, which can suppress TSH release from the pituitary gland.[30,31]

In the absence of clinical suspicion for early onset of hypothyroidism, thyroid function is assessed 4 to 6 weeks after surgery. Interpretation can be misleading in cases whereby both TSH and free T4 are within the lower end of normal laboratory parameters. Preoperative thyroid function testing, if available, can be helpful for comparison.

Treatment

When thyrotroph compromise is suspected, TSH is no longer a reliable marker for adequate thyroid hormone replacement, even in patients with preexisting primary hypothyroidism.[27,32] FT4 levels are more reflective of adequate thyroid hormone replacement after surgery, and normal TSH levels may actually suggest inadequate replacement.[32] At the authors' institution, FT4 levels, in the absence of other contraindications, are maintained toward the middle to upper limit of normal of the respective reference laboratory.[33,34] Levothyroxine may be started at a low dose of 25 μg per day and titrated up by increments of 25 μg to reach full replacement dose of 1.6 μg/kg/d, if needed, to maintain FT4 in the middle to upper limit of normal.[35,36] The effectiveness of thyroid hormone replacement is assessed at 6 weeks and 3 months after surgery to ensure adequate replacement and periodically thereafter.

Thyroid-stimulating hormone secreting tumors

Functional thyrotroph adenomas are rare, representing only 0.85% to 2.8% of all pituitary adenomas.[37] Perioperative management of hyperthyroidism includes radioactive iodine, β-blockers, and antithyroid medications, such as methimazole, thyroidectomy, or somatostatin analogues. Surgery is considered first-line treatment and achieves remission in 60% of macroadenomas, and normalization of, thyroid function and in 58% to 75% of cases. However, complete surgical cure is reported in only 40% of cases.[38] When surgery is not possible or there is recurrent unresectable disease, somatostatin analogues have shown benefit in normalizing thyroid hormonal levels, reducing goiter size, and reducing tumor size.[39,40]

Gonadal Axis

The incidence of new onset gonadal dysfunction after surgery is reported to be 1% to 5%.[1,3] If gonadotroph dysfunction is present before surgery, recovery occurs in 16% to 22% of nonfunctional adenomas without elevated prolactin due to stalk compression.[1,3] Many patients continue to have hypogonadotropic hypogonadism, even after resection of tumor, with hormonal replacement therapy dependent on a variety of factors.

Postoperative evaluation

For patients with preexisting hypogonadism on treatment, hormonal replacement can be continued in the perioperative setting. Typical postoperative hormonal assessment includes follicle stimulating hormone (FSH) and luteinizing hormone (LH) in addition to end-organ hormones, estradiol in women and testosterone in men, several weeks after surgery. Low or inappropriately normal LH and FSH in the setting of low testosterone or estradiol are suggestive of hypogonadotropic hypogonadism.[41] In premenopausal women, return or maintenance of menstrual cycles is often reflective of intact hypothalamic pituitary gonadal axis. Men should be screened with fasting morning testosterone, with demonstration of low testosterone on at least 2 separate occasions.[42]

Treatment

Women In premenopausal women, hormonal replacement is important for endometrial renewal, osteoporosis prevention, and cardiovascular protection. Various oral, vaginal, and transdermal formulations are commercially available. In early postmenopausal women, there should be a discussion regarding the risks and benefits of hormonal replacement therapy and should be individualized based on patient's symptoms and other risk factors.[43,44] Hormone replacement is generally not recommended in women over the age of 60, 10 years after menopause, or those with elevated risk of cardiovascular disease.[43,45]

Men In men who have symptoms of hypogonadism with biochemical confirmation, testosterone replacement should be initiated.[46] Several formulations are available, and replacement should aim for amelioration of hypogonadal symptoms and maintenance of secondary sex characteristics.[46] In older men, there is generally a natural decline in testosterone production with age.[47,48] Replacement with testosterone in older men, especially those without overt symptoms, is controversial.[47–49]

Growth Hormone Axis

Preoperative growth hormone deficiency (GHD) affects 30% to 41% of patients who undergo pituitary surgery, even with otherwise preserved pituitary function.[1,50] The likelihood of GHD also increases in the presence of other pituitary hormonal deficiencies.[50] Approximately 10% of patents recover function after surgery, whereas 6% of patients experience a new deficit.[1–3] GHD can occur in up to 60% of patients cured for acromegaly, and patients may require replacement.[51]

Postoperative evaluation of growth hormone deficiency

At the authors' institution, they assess for GHD approximately 6 weeks after surgery. A low insulin-like growth factor-1 (IGF-1) lower than 2 standard deviations below the age-matched mean has a 95% positive predictive value for GHD; however, many patients with GHD will have normal IGF-1 levels, and provocative testing can be especially helpful in these cases.[50,52,53] The insulin tolerance test (ITT) is considered a gold standard, but it is contraindicated in patients with cardiovascular disease, history of seizures, and the elderly. Safe administration requires close monitoring in an experienced center, with only a small portion of patients currently undergoing ITT.[50,54,55] Glucagon stimulation test is more commonly used and is considered a safe and reliable alternative to ITT.[56,57] Arginine growth hormone releasing hormone (GHRH) tests were used previously, but GHRH is no longer commercially available in the United States and may give false results in cases of GHD because of hypothalamic damage.[58,59] Arginine-levadopa stimulation test results are noted to be relatively less robust.[60,61] Most recently, oral Macimorelin (Macrilin; Aeterna Zentaris), a ghrelin receptor agonist that stimulates growth hormone release,

has shown promising results that are comparable to both the arginine-GHRH stimulation test and ITT.[62,63]

Treatment

Growth hormone (GH) replacement therapy for younger patients (<60 years old), can be initially started on 0.2 to 0.3 mg/d, whereas older patients may be started on 0.1 to 0.2 mg/d.[64] Data suggest patients with GHD who are replaced with GH have an improvement in quality-of-life, cardiovascular, and metabolic profiles, and bone health.[65–67] GH therapy is contraindicated in cases of active malignancy, but there is no consensus on timing of treatment even after remission.[64] Caution should also be used in patients with underlying diabetes mellitus (DM) or who develop DM during therapy.[64]

Acromegaly

Acromegaly is caused by a GH-secreting pituitary tumor, resulting in supranormal levels of circulating IGF-1 with associated metabolic and physiologic changes. Within hours after resection of GH-secreting adenomas, soft tissue swelling and metabolic parameters start to improve. Outcome is associated with smaller adenoma size, experience of surgeon, and preoperative GH level.[68] However, more recent evidence suggests that cure rates are relatively high, approaching 74% in some series.[69]

Postoperative evaluation

At the authors' institution, postoperative day 1 and day 2 GH levels are obtained. GH values less than 1 ng/mL in patients not previously treated with somatostatin analogues are prognostic of remission, although levels greater than 1 ng/mL are not necessarily a negative predictor of remission.[5,70,71] Three months after surgery, the authors reassess response to surgical therapy with IGF-1 levels and oral glucose tolerance test (OGTT); a corresponding GH less than 1.0 ng/mL and normal IGF-1 suggest an excellent response.[72] Periodic monitoring is recommended thereafter.

Treatment

In cases where remission is not possible or there is recurrence based on biochemical or imaging assessments, additional treatments may include somatostatin analogues, pegvisomant (GH antagonist), dopamine agonists, or radiation in surgically and medically refractory cases. Generally, repeat surgery is recommended for surgically amenable disease or residual tumor that is compressing vital structures. Medical therapy is recommended for patients with abnormal IGF-1 and moderate symptoms of excessive GH for whom surgical therapy is not indicated. An initial trial with a somatostatin analogue, pegvisomant, or somatostatin analogue in combination with pegvisomant for difficult-to-control disease may be used.[73,74] In patients who have minimal biochemical abnormalities with modest symptoms, cabergoline, a dopamine agonist, has shown benefit.[75]

Prolactin Axis

Surgery may be suitable for prolactinomas resistant to dopamine agonist therapy or those who develop cerebrospinal fluid leak. Surgical success is inversely related to serum prolactin levels and tumor size.[76] Microprolactinomas are particularly amenable to surgery with a cure rate of more than 70%, whereas macroprolactinomas demonstrate normalization of prolactin levels in only 32% of patients and a 19% recurrence rate.[77,78]

Postoperative evaluation

For those who undergo surgery, a postoperative day 1 prolactin level of less than 10 ng/mL is an excellent predictor of biochemical remission.[79] Prolactin levels can be reassessed 6 weeks after surgery, with normalization of prolactin levels usually reflective of remission or cure. Prolactin levels are followed closely for the first year after surgery; increasing levels may suggest recurrence or increasing tumor burden in cases where residual tumor remains. In patients with hyperprolactinemia owing to stalk compression, the vast majority have reported normalization of prolactin levels after surgery, with 100% improvement in galactorrhea, and 66.6% improvement in sexual function in a series of 267 patients.[80]

The most common hormonal deficiency associated with hyperprolactinemia is hypogonadotropic hypogonadism, because of suppression of gonadotrophs.[81] With postoperative normalization of prolactin levels, hypogonadal symptoms often resolve or mitigate. In premenopausal women, return of normal menses and resolution of galactorrhea are often an excellent clinical indicator of normal prolactin levels. In men, symptoms of hypogonadism, if present, should also resolve.

Treatment

If tumor remains, prolactin elevations may persist and may need to be medically managed with dopamine agonists or in certain cases treated with repeat surgery, or radiation. Radiation is generally reserved for patients who have failed surgical cure and are resistant to dopamine agonists, with normalization of prolactin only achieved in 50% of patients after 7.3 years.[82] Temozolomide, an alkylating agent, may also be effective in refractory cases.[83,84]

SUMMARY

As abnormalities in HPA hormones are frequent following surgery, evaluation and monitoring of hormones are critical. Appropriate management can have a profound effect on postsurgical morbidity, mortality, and long-term surgical success rates.

REFERENCES

1. Fatemi N, Dusick JR, Mattozo C, et al. Pituitary hormonal loss and recovery after transsphenoidal adenoma removal. Neurosurgery 2008;63(4):709–18 [discussion: 718–9].
2. Webb SM, Rigla M, Wagner A, et al. Recovery of hypopituitarism after neurosurgical treatment of pituitary adenomas. J Clin Endocrinol Metab 1999; 84(10):3696–700.
3. Jahangiri A, Wagner JR, Han SW, et al. Improved versus worsened endocrine function after transsphenoidal surgery for nonfunctional pituitary adenomas: rate, time course, and radiological analysis. J Neurosurg 2016;124(3):589–95.
4. Greenman Y, Tordjman K, Kisch E, et al. Relative sparing of anterior pituitary function in patients with growth hormone-secreting macroadenomas: comparison with nonfunctioning macroadenomas. J Clin Endocrinol Metab 1995;80(5):1577–83.
5. Woodmansee WW, Carmichael J, Kelly D, et al. American Association of Clinical Endocrinologists and American College of Endocrinology disease state clinical review: postoperative management following pituitary surgery. Endocr Pract 2015; 21(7):832–8.
6. Marko NF, Hamrahian AH, Weil RJ. Immediate postoperative cortisol levels accurately predict postoperative hypothalamic-pituitary-adrenal axis function after transsphenoidal surgery for pituitary tumors. Pituitary 2010;13(3):249–55.
7. Wentworth JM, Gao N, Sumithran KP, et al. Prospective evaluation of a protocol for reduced glucocorticoid replacement in transsphenoidal pituitary adenomectomy: prophylactic glucocorticoid replacement is seldom necessary. Clin Endocrinol (Oxf) 2008;68(1):29–35.
8. Rajaratnam S, Seshadri MS, Chandy MJ, et al. Hydrocortisone dose and postoperative diabetes insipidus in patients undergoing transsphenoidal pituitary surgery: a prospective randomized controlled study. Br J Neurosurg 2003;17(5):437–42.
9. Regan J, Watson J. Selective use of peri-operative steroids in pituitary tumor surgery: escape from dogma. Front Endocrinol (Lausanne) 2013;4:30.
10. Okinaga H, Matsuno A, Okazaki R. High risk of osteopenia and bone derangement in postsurgical

patients with craniopharyngiomas, pituitary adenomas and other parasellar lesions. Endocr J 2005;52(6):751–6.

11. Zueger T, Kirchner P, Herren C, et al. Glucocorticoid replacement and mortality in patients with nonfunctioning pituitary adenoma. J Clin Endocrinol Metab 2012;97(10):E1938–42.

12. Carosi G, Malchiodi E, Ferrante E, et al. Hypothalamic-pituitary axis in non-functioning pituitary adenomas: focus on the prevalence of isolated central hypoadrenalism. Neuroendocrinology 2015;102(4): 267–73.

13. Karavitaki N, Brufani C, Warner JT, et al. Craniopharyngiomas in children and adults: systematic analysis of 121 cases with long-term follow-up. Clin Endocrinol (Oxf) 2005;62(4):397–409.

14. Munro V, Tugwell B, Doucette S, et al. Recovery of adrenal function after chronic secondary adrenal insufficiency in patients with hypopituitarism. Clin Endocrinol (Oxf) 2016;85(2):216–22.

15. Burgers AM, Kokshoorn NE, Pereira AM, et al. Low incidence of adrenal insufficiency after transsphenoidal surgery in patients with acromegaly: a long-term follow-up study. J Clin Endocrinol Metab 2011;96(7):E1163–70.

16. Liamis G, Milionis HJ, Elisaf M. Endocrine disorders: causes of hyponatremia not to neglect. Ann Med 2011;43(3):179–87.

17. Salem M, Tainsh RE Jr, Bromberg J, et al. Perioperative glucocorticoid coverage. A reassessment 42 years after emergence of a problem. Ann Surg 1994;219(4):416–25.

18. McLaughlin N, Cohan P, Barnett P, et al. Early morning cortisol levels as predictors of short-term and long-term adrenal function after endonasal transsphenoidal surgery for pituitary adenomas and Rathke's cleft cysts. World Neurosurg 2013;80(5): 569–75.

19. Auchus RJ, Shewbridge RK, Shepherd MD. Which patients benefit from provocative adrenal testing after transsphenoidal pituitary surgery? Clin Endocrinol (Oxf) 1997;46(1):21–7.

20. Inder WJ, Hunt PJ. Glucocorticoid replacement in pituitary surgery: guidelines for perioperative assessment and management. J Clin Endocrinol Metab 2002;87(6):2745–50.

21. Dumont AS, Nemergut EC 2nd, Jane JA Jr, et al. Postoperative care following pituitary surgery. J Intensive Care Med 2005;20(3):127–40.

22. Alexandraki KI, Kaltsas GA, Isidori AM, et al. Long-term remission and recurrence rates in Cushing's disease: predictive factors in a single-centre study. Eur J Endocrinol 2013;168(4):639–48.

23. Acebes JJ, Martino J, Masuet C, et al. Early postoperative ACTH and cortisol as predictors of remission in Cushing's disease. Acta Neurochir (Wien) 2007;149(5):471–7 [discussion: 477–9].

24. Wagenmakers MA, Netea-Maier RT, van Lindert EJ, et al. Repeated transsphenoidal pituitary surgery (TS) via the endoscopic technique: a good therapeutic option for recurrent or persistent Cushing's disease (CD). Clin Endocrinol (Oxf) 2009;70(2): 274–80.

25. Nieman LK, Biller BM, Findling JW, et al. Treatment of Cushing's syndrome: an Endocrine Society Clinical Practice Guideline. J Clin Endocrinol Metab 2015;100(8):2807–31.

26. Gupta V, Lee M. Central hypothyroidism. Indian J Endocrinol Metab 2011;15(Suppl 2):S99–106.

27. Persani L, Ferretti E, Borgato S, et al. Circulating thyrotropin bioactivity in sporadic central hypothyroidism. J Clin Endocrinol Metab 2000;85(10): 3631–5.

28. Baajafer FS, Hammami MM, Mohamed GE. Prevalence and severity of hyponatremia and hypercreatininemia in short-term uncomplicated hypothyroidism. J Endocrinol Invest 1999;22(1):35–9.

29. Hammami MM, Almogbel F, Hammami S, et al. Acute severe hypothyroidism is not associated with hyponatremia even with increased water intake: a prospective study in thyroid cancer patients. BMC Endocr Disord 2013;13:27.

30. Haugen BR. Drugs that suppress TSH or cause central hypothyroidism. Best Pract Res Clin Endocrinol Metab 2009;23(6):793–800.

31. Wilber JF, Utiger RD. The effect of glucocorticoids on thyrotropin secretion. J Clin Invest 1969;48(11): 2096–103.

32. Shimon I, Cohen O, Lubetsky A, et al. Thyrotropin suppression by thyroid hormone replacement is correlated with thyroxine level normalization in central hypothyroidism. Thyroid 2002;12(9): 823–7.

33. Slawik M, Klawitter B, Meiser E, et al. Thyroid hormone replacement for central hypothyroidism: a randomized controlled trial comparing two doses of thyroxine (T4) with a combination of T4 and triiodothyronine. J Clin Endocrinol Metab 2007;92(11): 4115–22.

34. Iverson JF, Mariash CN. Optimal free thyroxine levels for thyroid hormone replacement in hypothyroidism. Endocr Pract 2008;14(5):550–5.

35. Ferretti E, Persani L, Jaffrain-Rea ML, et al. Evaluation of the adequacy of levothyroxine replacement therapy in patients with central hypothyroidism. J Clin Endocrinol Metab 1999;84(3):924–9.

36. Lania A, Persani L, Beck-Peccoz P. Central hypothyroidism. Pituitary 2008;11(2):181–6.

37. Mindermann T, Wilson CB. Thyrotropin-producing pituitary adenomas. J Neurosurg 1993;79(4):521–7.

38. Malchiodi E, Profka E, Ferrante E, et al. Thyrotropin-secreting pituitary adenomas: outcome of pituitary surgery and irradiation. J Clin Endocrinol Metab 2014;99(6):2069–76.

39. Socin HV, Chanson P, Delemer B, et al. The changing spectrum of TSH-secreting pituitary adenomas: diagnosis and management in 43 patients. Eur J Endocrinol 2003;148(4):433–42.

40. Bertherat J, Brue T, Enjalbert A, et al. Somatostatin receptors on thyrotropin-secreting pituitary adenomas: comparison with the inhibitory effects of octreotide upon in vivo and in vitro hormonal secretions. J Clin Endocrinol Metab 1992;75(2): 540 6.

41. Silveira LF, Latronico AC. Approach to the patient with hypogonadotropic hypogonadism. J Clin Endocrinol Metab 2013;98(5):1781–8.

42. Lamberts SW, de Herder WW, van der Lely AJ. Pituitary insufficiency. Lancet 1998;352(9122):127–34.

43. de Villiers TJ, Gass ML, Haines CJ, et al. Global Consensus Statement on menopausal hormone therapy. Maturitas 2013;74(4):391–2.

44. Anderson GL, Limacher M, Assaf AR, et al. Effects of conjugated equine estrogen in postmenopausal women with hysterectomy: the Women's Health Initiative randomized controlled trial. JAMA 2004; 291(14):1701–12.

45. Stuenkel CA, Gass ML, Manson JE, et al. A decade after the women's health initiative–the experts do agree. J Clin Endocrinol Metab 2012;97(8):2617–8.

46. Ponce OJ, Spencer-Bonilla G, Alvarez-Villalobos N, et al. The efficacy and adverse events of testosterone replacement therapy in hypogonadal men: a systematic review and meta-analysis of randomized, placebo-controlled trials. J Clin Endocrinol Metab 2018;103(5):1745–54.

47. Brawer MK. Testosterone replacement in men with andropause: an overview. Rev Urol 2004;6(Suppl 6):S9–15.

48. Cunningham GR. Andropause or male menopause? Rationale for testosterone replacement therapy in older men with low testosterone levels. Endocr Pract 2013;19(5):847–52.

49. Basaria S, Harman SM, Travison TG, et al. Effects of testosterone administration for 3 years on subclinical atherosclerosis progression in older men with low or low-normal testosterone levels: a randomized clinical trial. JAMA 2015;314(6):570–81.

50. Hartman ML, Crowe BJ, Biller BM, et al. Which patients do not require a GH stimulation test for the diagnosis of adult GH deficiency? J Clin Endocrinol Metab 2002;87(2):477–85.

51. Ronchi CL, Giavoli C, Ferrante E, et al. Prevalence of GH deficiency in cured acromegalic patients: impact of different previous treatments. Eur J Endocrinol 2009;161(1):37–42.

52. Hoffman DM, Nguyen TV, O'Sullivan AJ, et al. Diagnosis of growth hormone deficiency in adults. Lancet 1994;344(8920):482–3.

53. Svensson J, Johannsson G, Bengtsson BA. Insulin-like growth factor-I in growth hormone-deficient adults: relationship to population-based normal values, body composition and insulin tolerance test. Clin Endocrinol (Oxf) 1997;46(5):579–86.

54. Jones SL, Trainer PJ, Perry L, et al. An audit of the insulin tolerance test in adult subjects in an acute investigation unit over one year. Clin Endocrinol (Oxf) 1994;41(1):123–8.

55. Hoeck HC, Vestergaard P, Jakobsen PE, et al. Diagnosis of growth hormone (GH) deficiency in adults with hypothalamic-pituitary disorders: comparison of test results using pyridostigmine plus GH-releasing hormone (GHRH), clonidine plus GHRH, and insulin-induced hypoglycemia as GH secretagogues. J Clin Endocrinol Metab 2000;85(4): 1467–72.

56. Cain JP, Williams GH, Dluhy RG. Glucagon-initiated human growth hormone release: a comparative study. Can Med Assoc J 1972;107(7):617–22.

57. Berg C, Meinel T, Lahner H, et al. Diagnostic utility of the glucagon stimulation test in comparison to the insulin tolerance test in patients following pituitary surgery. Eur J Endocrinol 2010;162(3):477–82.

58. Darzy KH, Aimaretti G, Wieringa G, et al. The usefulness of the combined growth hormone (GH)-releasing hormone and arginine stimulation test in the diagnosis of radiation-induced GH deficiency is dependent on the post-irradiation time interval. J Clin Endocrinol Metab 2003; 88(1):95–102.

59. Bjork J, Link K, Erfurth EM. The utility of the growth hormone (GH) releasing hormone-arginine test for diagnosing GH deficiency in adults with childhood acute lymphoblastic leukemia treated with cranial irradiation. J Clin Endocrinol Metab 2005;90(11): 6048–54.

60. Biller BM, Grossman AB, Stewart PM, et al. Treatment of adrenocorticotropin-dependent Cushing's syndrome: a consensus statement. J Clin Endocrinol Metab 2008;93(7):2454–62.

61. Rahim A, Toogood AA, Shalet SM. The assessment of growth hormone status in normal young adult males using a variety of provocative agents. Clin Endocrinol (Oxf) 1996;45(5):557–62.

62. Garcia JM, Swerdloff R, Wang C, et al. Macimorelin (AEZS-130)-stimulated growth hormone (GH) test: validation of a novel oral stimulation test for the diagnosis of adult GH deficiency. J Clin Endocrinol Metab 2013;98(6):2422–9.

63. Garcia JM, Biller BMK, Korbonits M, et al. Macimorelin as a diagnostic test for adult GH deficiency. J Clin Endocrinol Metab 2018;103(8):3083–93.

64. Cook DM, Yuen KC, Biller BM, et al. American Association of Clinical Endocrinologists medical guidelines for clinical practice for growth hormone use in growth hormone-deficient adults and transition patients—2009 update. Endocr Pract 2009;15(Suppl 2):1–29.

65. Biermasz NR, Hamdy NA, Pereira AM, et al. Long-term skeletal effects of recombinant human growth hormone (rhGH) alone and rhGH combined with alendronate in GH-deficient adults: a seven-year follow-up study. Clin Endocrinol (Oxf) 2004;60(5): 568–75.

66. Bramnert M, Segerlantz M, Laurila E, et al. Growth hormone replacement therapy induces insulin resistance by activating the glucose-fatty acid cycle. J Clin Endocrinol Metab 2003;88(4): 1455–63.

67. Abs R, Bengtsson BA, Hernberg-Stahl E, et al. GH replacement in 1034 growth hormone deficient hypopituitary adults: demographic and clinical characteristics, dosing and safety. Clin Endocrinol (Oxf) 1999;50(6):703–13.

68. Barker FG 2nd, Klibanski A, Swearingen B. Transsphenoidal surgery for pituitary tumors in the United States, 1996-2000: mortality, morbidity, and the effects of hospital and surgeon volume. J Clin Endocrinol Metab 2003;88(10):4709–19.

69. Babu H, Ortega A, Nuno M, et al. Long-term endocrine outcomes following endoscopic endonasal transsphenoidal surgery for acromegaly and associated prognostic factors. Neurosurgery 2017;81(2): 357–66.

70. Krieger MD, Couldwell WT, Weiss MH. Assessment of long-term remission of acromegaly following surgery. J Neurosurg 2003;98(4):719–24.

71. Dutta P, Korbonits M, Sachdeva N, et al. Can immediate postoperative random growth hormone levels predict long-term cure in patients with acromegaly? Neurol India 2016;64(2):252–8.

72. Giustina A, Chanson P, Kleinberg D, et al. Expert consensus document: a consensus on the medical treatment of acromegaly. Nat Rev Endocrinol 2014; 10(4):243–8.

73. Trainer PJ, Ezzat S, D'Souza GA, et al. A randomized, controlled, multicentre trial comparing pegvisomant alone with combination therapy of pegvisomant and long-acting octreotide in patients with acromegaly. Clin Endocrinol (Oxf) 2009;71(4):549–57.

74. Madsen M, Poulsen PL, Orskov H, et al. Cotreatment with pegvisomant and a somatostatin analog (SA) in SA-responsive acromegalic patients. J Clin Endocrinol Metab 2011;96(8):2405–13.

75. Sandret L, Maison P, Chanson P. Place of cabergoline in acromegaly: a meta-analysis. J Clin Endocrinol Metab 2011;96(5):1327–35.

76. Tyrrell JB, Lamborn KR, Hannegan LT, et al. Transsphenoidal microsurgical therapy of prolactinomas: initial outcomes and long-term results. Neurosurgery 1999;44(2):254–61 [discussion: 261–53].

77. Serri O, Rasio E, Beauregard H, et al. Recurrence of hyperprolactinemia after selective transsphenoidal adenomectomy in women with prolactinoma. N Engl J Med 1983;309(5):280–3.

78. Donegan D, Atkinson JL, Jentoft M, et al. Surgical outcomes of prolactinomas in recent era: results of a heterogenous group. Endocr Pract 2017;23(1): 37–45.

79. Amar AP, Couldwell WT, Chen JC, et al. Predictive value of serum prolactin levels measured immediately after transsphenoidal surgery. J Neurosurg 2002;97(2):307–14.

80. Zaidi HA, Cote DJ, Castlen JP, et al. Time course of resolution of hyperprolactinemia after transsphenoidal surgery among patients presenting with pituitary stalk compression. World Neurosurg 2017;97:2–7.

81. Tolis G. Prolactin: physiology and pathology. Hosp Pract 1980;15(2):85–95.

82. Tsagarakis S, Grossman A, Plowman PN, et al. Megavoltage pituitary irradiation in the management of prolactinomas: long-term follow-up. Clin Endocrinol (Oxf) 1991;34(5):399–406.

83. Neff LM, Weil M, Cole A, et al. Temozolomide in the treatment of an invasive prolactinoma resistant to dopamine agonists. Pituitary 2007;10(1):81–6.

84. Fadul CE, Kominsky AL, Meyer LP, et al. Long-term response of pituitary carcinoma to temozolomide. Report of two cases. J Neurosurg 2006;105(4): 621–6.

Medical Management of Cushing Disease

Nicholas A. Tritos, MD, DSc*, Beverly M.K. Biller, MD

KEYWORDS

- Cabergoline • Cushing disease • Etomidate • Ketoconazole • Levoketoconazole • Metyrapone
- Mifepristone • Mltotane

KEY POINTS

- Medical therapy has an adjunctive role in the management of Cushing disease.
- Current treatment options include steroidogenesis inhibitors, centrally acting agents, and glucocorticoid receptor antagonists.
- Novel therapies currently in development may expand treatment options for Cushing disease.

INTRODUCTION

Transsphenoidal pituitary surgery (TSS) is the treatment of choice for the vast majority of patients with Cushing disease (CD) and can mitigate excess mortality in this patient population.[1–3] However, a high degree of neurosurgical expertise is required to optimize patient outcomes.[4]

Medical therapy is used adjunctively in patients with CD, including those who have failed TSS or who have experienced a postoperative recurrence and are not candidates for additional pituitary surgery.[5] In these patients, medical therapy is generally used in conjunction with radiation therapy to the sella with a goal toward controlling hypercortisolism until the beneficial effects of radiation therapy occur.[5,6] In some cases, medical therapy is used to control hypercortisolism preoperatively, including patients with severe symptoms and/or exuberant cortisol excess, in those who do not have ready access to an experienced neurosurgeon, patients whose tumor location is uncertain and, very rarely, those who decline surgery.[5,6]

Steroidogenesis inhibitors (ketoconazole, metyrapone, mitotane, etomidate), centrally acting agents (cabergoline, pasireotide, pasireotide LAR, temozolomide) and glucocorticoid receptor (GR) antagonists (mifepristone) are currently available for use as therapies in CD (**Tables 1** and **2**). Of note, most agents that are currently used in the United States are prescribed "off label" in patients with CD; only pasireotide, pasireotide LAR, and mifepristone are approved by the US Food and Drug Administration (FDA) for use in certain subsets of patients with hypercortisolism. Several compounds are at various stages of either clinical or preclinical development. As our understanding of the molecular underpinnings of these tumors improves, it is likely that novel targets will be identified and used to devise more effective therapeutic agents.

To identify the studies cited in this review article, electronic literature searches were conducted using the keywords "Cushing disease," "hypercortisolism," "medical therapy," "ketoconazole," "levoketoconazole," "metyrapone," "osilodrostat," "mitotane," "etomidate," "cabergoline," "pasireotide," "temozolomide," and "mifepristone." Articles were included in the present article at the authors' discretion.

Disclosure Statement: B.M.K. Biller has received institution-directed research support from Novartis and Strongbridge Biopharma and has consulted for Novartis and Strongbridge Biopharma. N.A. Tritos has received institution-directed research support from Ipsen and Novartis and has consulted for Strongbridge Biopharma.
Neuroendocrine Unit, Neuroendocrine and Pituitary Tumor Clinical Center, Massachusetts General Hospital, Harvard Medical School, 100 Blossom Street, Cox 1, Suite 140, Boston, MA 02114, USA
* Corresponding author.
E-mail address: ntritos@mgh.harvard.edu

Table 1
Steroidogenesis inhibitors used to treat hypercortisolism

Name	Dose Range	Effectiveness	Safety	Remarks
Ketoconazole	200–600 mg PO bid–tid	24 h UFC normalization in 49% of cases; escape may occur	Gastrointestinal toxicity, pruritus, transaminitis, severe hepatotoxicity	Regular monitoring of liver chemistries is advisable; gastric acid required for absorption; potential for drug-drug interactions
Metyrapone	250–1000 mg PO qid	Serum cortisol control in 76%; 24 h UFC normalization in 43%; escape may occur	Gastrointestinal upset, dizziness, hyperandrogenism (hirsutism, acne), mineralocorticoid excess (hypertension, edema, hypokalemia)	Most commonly used agent during pregnancy
Mitotane	0.5–3.0 g PO tid	24 h UFC normalization in up to 85%	Gastrointestinal, hepatic, metabolic, neurologic, hematologic, ophthalmic, skin, and bladder adverse effects	Abortifacient and teratogenic; delayed onset of action; used primarily in patients with adrenocortical carcinoma
Etomidate	0.03 mg/kg IV (bolus), followed by continuous infusion (0.1–0.3 mg/kg/h)	Highly effective in the short term; serum cortisol is helpful in monitoring	Sedation, nausea, vomiting, myoclonus, dystonia	Useful in severely ill inpatients as a bridge to other interventions; requires careful monitoring to avoid excessive sedation

All agents can induce hypoadrenalism as an extension of their pharmacologic action. None of the agents listed in this table are specifically approved for use in patients with CD in the United States.

Abbreviations: bid, twice daily; IV, intravenously; PO, orally; qid, 4 times daily; tid, 3 times daily; UFC, urine free cortisol.

STEROIDOGENESIS INHIBITORS

Several steroidogenesis inhibitors are currently available in the United States, including ketoconazole, metyrapone, mitotane, and etomidate (see **Table 1**), which are all used "off label" in patients with CD (ketoconazole and metyrapone are licensed by the European Medicines Agency for use in hypercortisolism). These pharmaceutic agents act on the adrenal cortex by inhibiting one or more enzymes involved in cortisol biosynthesis and thus have the potential to cause hypoadrenalism as an extension of their primary mechanism of action.[5,7,8] They are usually titrated toward normalizing 24-hour urine free cortisol (UFC). Alternatively, these drugs can be used to completely inhibit cortisol secretion while exogenous glucocorticoid replacement is being administered in a "block-and-replace" regimen. This latter approach can be particularly helpful in patients

with cyclic hypercortisolism. Of note, escape (tachyphylaxis) from the salutary effects of these agents may occur in some cases, thus necessitating close patient follow-up.

Ketoconazole is an imidazole derivative that is FDA approved as an antibiotic for fungal infections. In addition to its antifungal properties, ketoconazole inhibits multiple enzymes involved in adrenal steroidogenesis. Ketoconazole has been studied in several case series of patients with Cushing syndrome (CS) of diverse etiology, including those with CD.[9,10] In a recently published retrospective analysis of 200 patients with hypercortisolism who were treated with ketoconazole as monotherapy at 14 centers in France, ketoconazole therapy led to 24-hour UFC normalization in 49% of cases.[11] Blood pressure, glucose, and potassium levels also improved in treated patients.

Table 2
Centrally acting agents used in patients with Cushing disease

Name	Dose Range	Effectiveness	Safety	Remarks
Cabergoline	0.5–7.0 mg PO weekly	24 h UFC normalization in up to 40% of cases; escape may occur	Nausea, orthostatic dizziness, headache, nasal congestion, psychiatric manifestations, (?) valvulopathy	Effective doses are higher than those typically used in hyperprolactinemia
Pasireotide	0.3–0.9 mg SC bid	24 h UFC normalization in up to 26% of cases; escape seems uncommon	Gastrointestinal toxicity, gallstones, hypoadrenalism, hyperglycemia/ diabetes mellitus, QT prolongation	Glucose monitoring is needed
Pasireotide LAR	10–30 mg IM every 4 wk	24 h UFC normalization in 41% of cases	Gastrointestinal toxicity, gallstones, hypoadrenalism, hyperglycemia/ diabetes mellitus, QT prolongation	Glucose monitoring is needed
Temozolomide	150–200 mg/m²/d PO for 5 d each month	Partial or complete tumor response in up to 80% of cases; escape may occur	Neutropenia, thrombocytopenia, gastrointestinal toxicity, headache, dizziness, hearing loss	Administered by a neuro-oncologist; used in patients with aggressive tumors refractory to other interventions

Only pasireotide and pasireotide LAR are specifically approved for use in patients with CD.
Abbreviations: bid, twice daily; IM, intramuscularly; PO, orally; SC, subcutaneously; UFC, urine free cortisol.

About 20% of patients discontinued ketoconazole because of intolerance, including hypoadrenalism, pruritus, and gastrointestinal side effects. Abnormalities in liver chemistries, including elevations in serum aminotransferase levels, were noted in 18% of patients and were severe (exceeding 5 times the upper limit of normal) in 2.5% of cases.[11]

In most patients, transaminitis is asymptomatic and reversible on ketoconazole withdrawal or dose reduction, which is advisable when serum aminotransferase levels exceed 3 times the upper limit of their reference range. On the other hand, severe, potentially life-threatening hepatotoxicity has been reported in approximately 1 in 15,000 patients treated with ketoconazole.[12] The FDA has inserted a "black-box warning" into the ketoconazole prescribing information to alert patients and physicians of the drug's potential for serious hepatic injury, and recommends frequent laboratory monitoring of treated patients. Other possible adverse effects include headache, gynecomastia, and hypogonadism in men; the latter 2 occur as a consequence of inhibition of testosterone biosynthesis. As a corollary, ketoconazole has the potential to interfere with masculinization of a male fetus. It is therefore prudent to avoid ketoconazole use during pregnancy.

Ketoconazole requires gastric acid for absorption. As a consequence, the drug is poorly absorbed in patients with achlorhydria or those who take medications that decrease gastric acidity. In addition, ketoconazole has the potential for drug-drug interactions with other agents metabolized by enzymes of the cytochrome P450 3A4 (CYP3A4) hepatic system.[5,8] Careful attention to concurrently prescribed medications is required to avoid potentially serious interactions with ketoconazole.

Metyrapone, another steroidogenesis inhibitor, exerts its salutary effects on cortisol secretion by primarily inhibiting 11β-hydroxylase, the terminal enzyme involved in cortisol synthesis.[13] It has a rapid onset of action, which can be particularly helpful when prompt control of hypercortisolism is required in an outpatient setting. In metyrapone-treated patients, cortisol levels should be assayed using techniques that can distinguish between cortisol and its precursors, including 11-deoxycortisol, which accumulate during metyrapone therapy.

A recently published study retrospectively reported on the outcomes of 195 patients with hypercortisolism (including 115 patients with CD) who were treated with metyrapone at 13 centers in the United Kingdom.[14] The drug was used as monotherapy in 164 cases. Control of hypercortisolism was achieved in 76% of patients based on serum cortisol levels and 43% based on 24-hour UFC.

Adverse events were reported in 25% of patients, including dizziness and gastrointestinal upset, and were reversible with dose adjustments.[14] Other adverse events associated with metyrapone use include hyperandrogenism in women (hirsutism, acne) and mineralocorticoid excess (hypertension, edema, hypokalemia), which occur as a consequence of accumulation of steroid precursors with androgenic or mineralocorticoid activity, respectively. Monitoring of blood pressure, serum potassium, and testosterone levels is advisable in treated patients.[5,8]

Metyrapone has been used successfully to control hypercortisolism during pregnancy.[15] However, it does not carry a specific FDA-approved indication for use during gestation.[16]

Mitotane (o,p'-DDD) is chemically related to an insecticide (dichlorodiphenyltrichloroethane [DDT]). In addition to inhibiting several steps in adrenal steroidogenesis, mitotane is adrenolytic, particularly when administered in higher doses over several months. Mitotane has been FDA approved for use in patients with adrenocortical carcinoma.[17–19] Retrospectively collected data from Europe suggest that mitotane administration leads to 24-hour UFC normalization in 70% to 85% of patients with CD.[20] However, it is rarely used in patients with CD in the United States.

Mitotane has a slow onset of action (several weeks) and is therefore not suitable as monotherapy when rapid control of hypercortisolism is desirable. As hypoadrenalism is generally anticipated to develop, patients treated with mitotane should receive glucocorticoid replacement. Mitotane administration accelerates glucocorticoid metabolism and increases corticosteroid-binding globulin levels. As a consequence, patients treated with mitotane generally require a higher than usual glucocorticoid replacement dose. Mitotane is extensively stored in adipose tissue and is slowly eliminated after drug discontinuation. It is also abortifacient and teratogenic, and should not be used during gestation. As a consequence, it is advisable to avoid pregnancy for 5 years after mitotane discontinuation.[5,8]

Mitotane use is associated with several potential adverse effects, including gastrointestinal, hepatic, metabolic, neurologic, hematologic, ophthalmic, skin, and bladder toxicities, which may limit its clinical utility.

Etomidate is the only agent that is currently available for intravenous administration in patients with CS of diverse etiology, including CD.[21–24] It is licensed as an anesthetic but has also been found to have useful activity in patients with hypercortisolism, wherein it acts by inhibiting 11β-hydroxylase, even in subhypnotic doses. After intravenous administration, etomidate leads to a rapid decrease (within hours) in serum cortisol levels.[21–24] It can be particularly helpful in patients with severe hypercortisolism who require a "bridge" to definitive therapy.[25] Etomidate use requires careful dose titration and patient monitoring in the intensive care unit to avoid excessive sedation.[25] Other potential adverse effects may include nausea, vomiting, myoclonus, and dystonia.

Several steroidogenesis inhibitors are currently in development, including levoketoconazole, osilodrostat, abiraterone, and ATR-101. Levoketoconazole is a ketoconazole enantiomer (2S,4R) that is being studied as a possible therapy in patients with CS (including those with CD). Preclinical data have suggested that levoketoconazole is more potent than its enantiomer (2R,4S) in inhibiting the activity of several enzymes involved in adrenal steroidogenesis while having a lower potential to induce hepatic inflammation.[26] An open-label clinical trial was conducted to evaluate the efficacy and safety of levoketoconazole in patients with CS, including those with CD (https://clinicaltrials.gov/: NCT01838551), but the results have not yet been published, and a phase 3 double-blind, randomized study of levoketoconazole with a placebo arm is under way (https://clinicaltrials.gov/: NCT03277690).

Osilodrostat, another investigational agent, inhibits 11β-hydroxylase and aldosterone synthase. In a phase 2 study, osilodrostat administration led to 24-hour UFC normalization in 92% of 12 patients with CD.[27] In a longer (22-week) study, 79% of 19 patients normalized their 24-hour UFC.[28] Phase 3 studies of osilodrostat (https://clinicaltrials.gov/: NCT02468193 and NCT02697734) are being conducted and are anticipated to yield data that may establish whether escape from the effects of osilodrostat can occur with long-term use. Adverse events reported thus far include headache, nausea, dizziness, arthralgias, and androgenic (hirsutism, acne), and mineralocorticoid (hypertension, edema, hypokalemia) effects.

Abiraterone acetate is an inhibitor of 17α-hydroxylase and 17,20-lyase that has been efficacious in patients with metastatic prostate carcinoma by means of decreasing testosterone synthesis.[29,30] In a case study, a patient with severe hypercortisolism secondary to adrenocortical carcinoma showed a short-term response to abiraterone acetate.[31] Following encouraging preclinical data,[32] a study of abiraterone acetate in patients with adrenocortical carcinoma is under way (https://clinicaltrials.gov/ NCT03145285). There are no clinical data on patients with CD treated with abiraterone acetate.

ATR-101 is a small molecule that inhibits acyl coenzyme A:cholesterol acyltransferase 1 (ACAT1), which catalyzes the esterification of cholesterol into cholesterol esters, an important starting point in the biosynthesis of adrenal steroids. ATR-101 administration to dogs with CS led to a significant decrease in cortisol levels.[33] A phase 2 study of ATR-101 in patients with CD is under way (https://clinicaltrials.gov/: NCT03053271).

Efforts are also being made to devise effective strategies aimed at inhibiting adrenocorticotropin (ACTH) signaling, including a monoclonal antibody (ALD1613) that neutralizes ACTH, and peptide antagonists of the melanocortin-2 receptor, which mediates ACTH action.[26,34] Clinical data involving use of these compounds in patients with CD are currently lacking.

CENTRALLY ACTING AGENTS

These medications act by inhibiting ACTH secretion on tumorous corticotrophs, leading to a decrease in 24-hour UFC (see **Table 2**). Cabergoline, pasireotide, and pasireotide LAR are currently available for use in patients with CD in the United States. Temozolomide is also used "off label" in patients with aggressive pituitary tumors.

Cabergoline is a D2-selective dopamine receptor agonist, which has been approved by the FDA for use in patients with hyperprolactinemia[35]; its use in patients with CD is "off label." The effectiveness of cabergoline in CD is predicated by the presence of D2 receptors in most corticotroph tumors.[36] There are no published randomized clinical trials of cabergoline administration in patients with CD. Several studies have reported that cabergoline therapy, administered in doses up to 7 mg/wk, leads to 24-hour UFC normalization in up to 40% of patients with CD.[37–39] However, escape from its beneficial effects may occur over time.

Cabergoline is well tolerated by most patients. On the other hand, adverse effects may occur among those on cabergoline therapy, including nausea and orthostatic dizziness, which may improve over time. Some adverse effects can be minimized by slow titration and administration with a snack at bedtime. Other adverse effects associated with cabergoline use include headache, nasal congestion, constipation, vivid

dreams, nightmares, anxiety, and depression. This medication should be avoided in patients with psychosis, who may experience an exacerbation of their symptoms on cabergoline therapy. In addition, manifestations of impulsivity may develop in a small number of treated patients.[35,40–43] Cabergoline discontinuation is advisable in patients who develop severe psychiatric symptoms.

Cardiac valvulopathy has been reported in patients with Parkinson's disease who received very high cabergoline doses, and may occur as a consequence of serotonin receptor activation in the endocardium.[44] A recent meta-analysis reported an increased risk of tricuspid regurgitation in patients with hyperprolactinemia treated with cabergoline.[45] However, this finding was essentially driven by observations made in a single study.[46] Whether cardiac valvulopathy might develop in patients with CD treated with cabergoline has not been established. It may be prudent to perform periodic cardiac echocardiograms in patients treated with higher cabergoline doses (>2 mg/wk). However, it should be noted that the cost-effectiveness of this strategy has not been determined.

Pasireotide and its long-acting formulation, pasireotide LAR, are somatostatin receptor (SSTR) agonists that activate multiple receptor isoforms, including SSTRs 1, 2, 3, and 5.[47] These receptors are present in most corticotroph adenomas.[36] In particular, it is thought that SSTR2 and SSTR5 receptor activation is important for efficacy in patients with CD.[47] In a phase 3 study, 162 patients with CD were randomly allocated to either of 2 doses of pasireotide (600 μg twice daily or 900 μg twice daily).[48] At 6 months, 15% of patients in the lower-dose group and 26% of patients in the higher-dose group normalized their 24-hour UFC. In addition, tumor volume reduction was noted in up to 44% of patients with measurable tumor size. Tachyphylaxis may occasionally occur among patients treated with pasireotide. In another phase 3 study, 150 patients with CD were randomized to pasireotide LAR at a starting dose of either 10 mg or 30 mg every 4 weeks and were treated over a 12-month period.[49] In this study, 24-hour UFC normalization (at 7 months) was reported in 41.9% of patients on the lower starting dose and 40.8% of those on the higher starting dose. In addition, beneficial effects on body weight, serum lipids, and blood pressure were reported in treated patients. Pasireotide LAR was reported to decrease tumor size in a patient with Nelson syndrome.[50] Both medications have been approved by the FDA for use in patients with CD who have failed pituitary surgery or are not surgical candidates.

Both pasireotide and pasireotide LAR are associated with the same gastrointestinal adverse effects that have been observed in patients treated with other somatostatin receptor agonists, including diarrhea, nausea, abdominal pain, and cholelithiasis.[48,49] Adrenal insufficiency, hair loss, vitamin B12 deficiency, asymptomatic sinus bradycardia, and QT prolongation may develop in a minority of treated patients. In addition, patients on either pasireotide or pasireotide LAR therapy often develop hyperglycemia (in 70% to 80% of cases) that may be severe enough to necessitate the institution of antihyperglycemic therapy.[48,49] The hyperglycemic effect of pasireotide/pasireotide LAR is a consequence of direct inhibition of insulin and incretin secretion.[51] Metformin, incretin-related therapies, and insulin have been proposed as preferred treatments of patients on pasireotide/pasireotide LAR therapy who develop hyperglycemia or diabetes mellitus.[5,8]

Temozolomide is an orally active alkylating agent that is approved by the FDA for treatment of some gliomas.[52] It causes DNA methylation at specific guanine (O^6) sites, thus interfering with DNA replication of dividing cells and inducing apoptosis. The repair enzyme O^6-methylguanine-DNA methyltransferase (MGMT) acts to reverse DNA damage induced by temozolomide. In some, but not all, studies lower MGMT activity has been associated with a better tumor response.[52] Temozolomide can induce a complete or partial tumor response in up to 80% of patients with CD and has been used "off label" in patients with aggressive corticotroph tumors.[52,53] However, escape from its salutary effects may occur over time. This medication is administered by a neuro-oncologist at a typical dose of 150 to 200 mg/m^2/d for 5 days each month. Adverse events include neutropenia, thrombocytopenia, gastrointestinal toxicity, headache, dizziness, and hearing loss.

Several investigational therapies are being studied as potential treatments in patients with CD. Retinoic acid activates its cognate receptors to inhibit pro-opiomelanocortin expression, ACTH secretion, and corticotroph tumor growth in preclinical studies.[54] Isotretinoin, a 13-*cis*-retinoic acid isomer, was efficacious in controlling hypercortisolism in approximately 25% of patients with CD in small studies.[55,56] Adequately powered clinical trials are required to fully establish the safety and efficacy of this potential therapy in CD.

Recent studies have identified somatic, activating mutations in the *ubiquitin-specific peptidase 8* (*USP8*) gene in 31% to 62% of corticotroph tumors.[57] Based on in vitro and animal data, *USP8* mutations likely promote both ACTH secretion and tumor growth by increasing the number of epidermal growth factor (EGF) receptors and upregulating downstream signaling pathways.[58] In preclinical studies, the tyrosine kinase inhibitor gefitinib, which has been approved for the treatment of non–small cell lung cancer with activating EGF receptor mutations, was found to inhibit ACTH secretion and tumor growth.[59] A phase 2 clinical study of gefitinib in patients with CD whose tumors bear *USP8* mutations is in progress (http://clinicaltrials.gov: NCT02484755).

R-roscovitine is an inhibitor of cyclin-dependent kinase 2 and cyclin E.[60] In animal studies, R-roscovitine decreased ACTH secretion and tumor growth.[61] A phase 2 clinical study of R-roscovitine in patients with CD is under way (http://clinicaltrials.gov: NCT02160730).

Silibinin binds to heat-shock protein 90 to promote its dissociation from the GR, thus enhancing GR action, including feedback inhibition of cortisol on tumorous corticotrophs.[62] Silibinin appears to be promising in both in vitro and animal studies, but clinical data in patients with CD are currently lacking.[62]

GLUCOCORTICOID RECEPTOR ANTAGONISTS

Mifepristone is a GR as well as progesterone receptor (PR) antagonist that is FDA approved for use in patients with CS (including those with CD) who have hyperglycemia and have either failed surgery or are not surgical candidates (**Table 3**).[63,64] In a phase 3 study, 50 patients with CS, including a majority of those with CD, who had either hyperglycemia or hypertension, received mifepristone therapy for 24 weeks in an open-label, forced dose titration protocol.[65] In this study, 60% of 29 patients with hyperglycemia or diabetes mellitus improved with regard to glucose tolerance. In addition, glycohemoglobin levels decreased from 7.4% to 6.3% and antihyperglycemic agents were decreased in 7 of 15 patients. In the subgroup of patients with hypertension, 38% of 21 patients improved with regard to blood pressure by at least 5 mm Hg. Overall, study patients showed a 5.7% decrease in body weight from baseline, and 87% of patients showed an improvement in global clinical status.[65]

Cortisol and ACTH levels increase from baseline in patients with CD during mifepristone therapy.[66] As a consequence, drug effectiveness must be established on clinical criteria at present. Similarly, hypoadrenalism, which can occur as a consequence of excessive GR blockade, must be recognized based on clinical grounds alone. Patients who experience symptoms suggestive

Table 3
Glucocorticoid receptor antagonist used in patients with Cushing syndrome/disease

Name	Dose Range	Effectiveness	Safety	Remarks
Mifepristone	300–1200 mg PO daily	Improvement in hyperglycemia in 60% of hyperglycemic or diabetic patients; decrease in blood pressure in 38% of hypertensive patients; global clinical improvement in 87% of cases	Hypoadrenalism, hypertension, hypokalemia, endometrial thickening/vaginal bleeding, elevations in serum thyrotropin and lipids	Treatment monitoring based only on clinical criteria at present; abortifacient; potential for drug-drug interactions

Mifepristone is FDA approved for patients with CS (including CD) who are hyperglycemic and are not candidates for surgery or have failed surgery.
Abbreviation: PO, orally.

of hypoadrenalism can be rescued by dexamethasone administration in higher than replacement doses administered over several days.

Patients treated with mifepristone may develop increases in blood pressure or hypokalemia as a consequence of unopposed cortisol interaction with the mineralocorticoid receptor. Regular monitoring of blood pressure and serum potassium levels is advisable. In addition to potassium replacement, spironolactone therapy can be helpful in patients who develop such sequelae of mineralocorticoid excess. Endometrial thickening and vaginal bleeding may develop in women as a consequence of PR inhibition; however, precancerous endometrial hyperplasia has not been reported. The drug will terminate pregnancy and is contraindicated in women during gestation.

Other adverse effects associated with mifepristone use include fatigue, headache, nausea, and reversible elevations in serum thyrotropin and lipids. Regular imaging of pituitary tumors is prudent because the drug has no direct antitumor effects and inhibits GR-mediated feedback; however, there have been no consistent findings to suggest that mifepristone therapy leads to an increase in tumor size despite increases in ACTH levels.[66] Mifepristone inhibits CYP3A4 and other hepatic enzymes and has the potential for interactions with other drugs metabolized through the same pathways. Therefore, it is important to review all concomitant medications for possible interactions with mifepristone.

Relacorilant (CORT125134) is a novel, investigational GR antagonist that does not interact with the PR.[26,67] Relacorilant was administered to 32 patients with CS (including those with CD) in a phase 2 open-label study, during which subjects were allocated to either of 2 dose groups and treated for 16 weeks (http://clinicaltrials.gov: NCT02804750). Preliminary findings from this study, including improvements in glycemic and blood pressure control, were presented at the 2018 American Association of Clinical Endocrinologists annual meeting.[68] A phase 3 study of relacorilant is under way (http://clinicaltrials.gov: NCT03697109). Based on its mechanism of action, it is anticipated that this compound may be unlikely to induce endometrial thickening or vaginal bleeding.

SUMMARY

Several medical therapy options exist to treat patients with CD, including steroidogenesis inhibitors, centrally acting agents, and GR antagonists. The choice between different agents is empiric, since no head-to-head clinical trials comparing different therapies have been published. Factors that may influence the choice between different medications include the severity of hypercortisolism and associated symptoms, the need for rapid disease control, tumor size, comorbidities, concurrent medications and potential for drug-drug interactions, patient experience with medical therapies, patient preference and ability to adhere to a complex medical regimen, and coverage of medical therapy by insurance carriers.

Combination therapies have been studied in case series, including ketoconazole plus metyrapone with or without mitotane, ketoconazole plus cabergoline, or cabergoline plus pasireotide and ketoconazole, and can be helpful in patients with severe hypercortisolism.[69–72] Larger clinical trials of adequate power and duration are needed to fully characterize the efficacy and safety of combination therapies in patients with CD.

Despite several advances in medical therapies, there are substantial unmet medical needs among patients with CD. Currently available therapeutic agents have an important, yet adjunctive, role in the management of hypercortisolism. It is anticipated that recent and future advances in our understanding of the molecular pathogenesis of corticotroph tumors will lead to further progress in the development of highly efficacious and safe therapeutic agents for this serious condition.

REFERENCES

1. Cushing H. The basophil adenomas of the pituitary body and their clinical manifestations (pituitary basophilism). Bull Johns Hopkins Hosp 1932;50: 137–95.
2. Cushing H. The basophil adenomas of the pituitary body. Ann R Coll Surg Engl 1969;44(4):180–1.
3. Swearingen B, Biller BM, Barker FG 2nd, et al. Long-term mortality after transsphenoidal surgery for Cushing disease. Ann Intern Med 1999;130(10): 821–4.
4. Barker FG 2nd, Klibanski A, Swearingen B. Transsphenoidal surgery for pituitary tumors in the United States, 1996-2000: mortality, morbidity, and the effects of hospital and surgeon volume. J Clin Endocrinol Metab 2003;88(10):4709–19.
5. Nieman LK, Biller BM, Findling JW, et al. Treatment of Cushing's syndrome: an Endocrine Society clinical practice guideline. J Clin Endocrinol Metab 2015;100(8):2807–31.
6. Tritos NA, Biller BM, Swearingen B. Management of Cushing disease. Nat Rev Endocrinol 2011;7(5): 279–89.
7. Nieman LK. Update in the medical therapy of Cushing's disease. Curr Opin Endocrinol Diabetes Obes 2013;20(4):330–4.
8. Tritos NA, Biller BM. Medical management of Cushing's disease. J Neurooncol 2014;117(3):407–14.
9. Sonino N, Boscaro M, Paoletta A, et al. Ketoconazole treatment in Cushing's syndrome: experience in 34 patients. Clin Endocrinol (Oxf) 1991;35(4): 347–52.
10. Tabarin A, Navarranne A, Guerin J, et al. Use of ketoconazole in the treatment of Cushing's disease and ectopic ACTH syndrome. Clin Endocrinol (Oxf) 1991;34(1):63–9.
11. Castinetti F, Guignat L, Giraud P, et al. Ketoconazole in Cushing's disease: is it worth a try? J Clin Endocrinol Metab 2014;99(5):1623–30.
12. McCance DR, Ritchie CM, Sheridan B, et al. Acute hypoadrenalism and hepatotoxicity after treatment with ketoconazole. Lancet 1987;1(8532):573.
13. Verhelst JA, Trainer PJ, Howlett TA, et al. Short and long-term responses to metyrapone in the medical management of 91 patients with Cushing's syndrome. Clin Endocrinol (Oxf) 1991;35(2):169–78.
14. Daniel E, Aylwin S, Mustafa O, et al. Effectiveness of metyrapone in treating Cushing's syndrome: a retrospective multicenter study in 195 patients. J Clin Endocrinol Metab 2015;100(11):4146–54.
15. Gormley MJ, Hadden DR, Kennedy TL, et al. Cushing's syndrome in pregnancy–treatment with metyrapone. Clin Endocrinol (Oxf) 1982;16(3):283–93.
16. Lindsay JR, Jonklaas J, Oldfield EH, et al. Cushing's syndrome during pregnancy: personal experience and review of the literature. J Clin Endocrinol Metab 2005;90(5):3077–83.
17. Luton JP, Cerdas S, Billaud L, et al. Clinical features of adrenocortical carcinoma, prognostic factors, and the effect of mitotane therapy. N Engl J Med 1990;322(17):1195–201.
18. Mauclere-Denost S, Leboulleux S, Borget I, et al. High-dose mitotane strategy in adrenocortical carcinoma: prospective analysis of plasma mitotane measurement during the first 3 months of follow-up. Eur J Endocrinol 2012;166(2):261–8.
19. Terzolo M, Angeli A, Fassnacht M, et al. Adjuvant mitotane treatment for adrenocortical carcinoma. N Engl J Med 2007;356(23):2372–80.
20. Baudry C, Coste J, Bou Khalil R, et al. Efficiency and tolerance of mitotane in Cushing's disease in 76 patients from a single center. Eur J Endocrinol 2012; 167(4):473–81.
21. Allolio B, Schulte HM, Kaulen D, et al. Nonhypnotic low-dose etomidate for rapid correction of hypercortisolaemia in Cushing's syndrome. Klin Wochenschr 1988;66(8):361–4.
22. Drake WM, Perry LA, Hinds CJ, et al. Emergency and prolonged use of intravenous etomidate to control hypercortisolemia in a patient with Cushing's syndrome and peritonitis. J Clin Endocrinol Metab 1998;83(10):3542–4.
23. Preda VA, Sen J, Karavitaki N, et al. Etomidate in the management of hypercortisolaemia in Cushing's syndrome: a review. Eur J Endocrinol 2012;167(2): 137–43.
24. Schulte HM, Benker G, Reinwein D, et al. Infusion of low dose etomidate: correction of hypercortisolemia in patients with Cushing's syndrome and dose-response relationship in normal subjects. J Clin Endocrinol Metab 1990;70(5):1426–30.
25. Carroll TB, Peppard WJ, Herrmann DJ, et al. Continuous etomidate infusion for the management of severe Cushing syndrome: validation of a standard protocol. J Endocr Soc 2019;3(1):1–12.
26. Cuevas-Ramos D, Lim DST, Fleseriu M. Update on medical treatment for Cushing's disease. Clin Diabetes Endocrinol 2016;2:16.
27. Bertagna X, Pivonello R, Fleseriu M, et al. LCI699, a potent 11beta-hydroxylase inhibitor, normalizes urinary cortisol in patients with Cushing's disease:

results from a multicenter, proof-of-concept study. J Clin Endocrinol Metab 2014;99(4):1375–83.

28. Fleseriu M, Pivonello R, Young J, et al. Osilodrostat, a potent oral 11beta-hydroxylase inhibitor: 22-week, prospective, Phase II study in Cushing's disease. Pituitary 2016;19(2):138–48.

29. Berruti A, Pia A, Terzolo M. Abiraterone and increased survival in metastatic prostate cancer. N Engl J Med 2011;365(8):766 [author reply: 767–8].

30. Gartrell BA, Saad F. Abiraterone in the management of castration-resistant prostate cancer prior to chemotherapy. Ther Adv Urol 2015;7(4):194–202.

31. Claps M, Lazzari B, Grisanti S, et al. Management of severe Cushing syndrome induced by adrenocortical carcinoma with abiraterone acetate: a case report. AACE Clin Case Rep 2016;2(4):e337–41.

32. Fiorentini C, Fragni M, Perego P, et al. Antisecretive and antitumor activity of abiraterone acetate in human adrenocortical cancer: a preclinical study. J Clin Endocrinol Metab 2016;101(12):4594–602.

33. Langlois DK, Fritz MC, Schall WD, et al. ATR-101, a selective ACAT1 inhibitor, decreases ACTH-stimulated cortisol concentrations in dogs with naturally occurring Cushing's syndrome. BMC Endocr Disord 2018;18(1):24.

34. Feldhaus AL, Anderson K, Dutzar B, et al. ALD1613, a novel long-acting monoclonal antibody to control ACTH-driven pharmacology. Endocrinology 2017; 158(1):1–8.

35. Klibanski A. Clinical practice. Prolactinomas. N Engl J Med 2010;362(13):1219–26.

36. de Bruin C, Feelders RA, Lamberts SW, et al. Somatostatin and dopamine receptors as targets for medical treatment of Cushing's syndrome. Rev Endocr Metab Disord 2009;10(2):91–102.

37. Godbout A, Manavela M, Danilowicz K, et al. Cabergoline monotherapy in the long-term treatment of Cushing's disease. Eur J Endocrinol 2010;163(5): 709–16.

38. Pivonello R, De Martino MC, Cappabianca P, et al. The medical treatment of Cushing's disease: effectiveness of chronic treatment with the dopamine agonist cabergoline in patients unsuccessfully treated by surgery. J Clin Endocrinol Metab 2009; 94(1):223–30.

39. Burman P, Eden-Engstrom B, Ekman B, et al. Limited value of cabergoline in Cushing's disease: a prospective study of a 6-week treatment in 20 patients. Eur J Endocrinol 2016;174(1):17–24.

40. Bancos I, Nannenga MR, Bostwick JM, et al. Impulse control disorders in patients with dopamine agonist-treated prolactinomas and nonfunctioning pituitary adenomas: a case-control study. Clin Endocrinol (Oxf) 2014;80(6):863–8.

41. Bancos I, Nippoldt TB, Erickson D. Hypersexuality in men with prolactinomas treated with dopamine agonists. Endocrine 2017;56(3):456–7.

42. Barake M, Evins AE, Stoeckel L, et al. Investigation of impulsivity in patients on dopamine agonist therapy for hyperprolactinemia: a pilot study. Pituitary 2014;17(2):150–6.

43. Barake M, Klibanski A, Tritos NA. MANAGEMENT OF ENDOCRINE DISEASE: impulse control disorders in patients with hyperpolactinemia treated with dopamine agonists: how much should we worry? Eur J Endocrinol 2018;179(6):R287–96.

44. Zanettini R, Antonini A, Gatto G, et al. Valvular heart disease and the use of dopamine agonists for Parkinson's disease. N Engl J Med 2007;356(1):39–46.

45. Stiles CE, Tetteh-Wayoe ET, Bestwick J, et al. A meta-analysis of the prevalence of cardiac valvulopathy in hyperprolactinemic patients treated with Cabergoline. J Clin Endocrinol Metab 2018. https:// doi.org/10.1210/jc.2018-01071. [Epub ahead of print].

46. Colao A, Galderisi M, Di Sarno A, et al. Increased prevalence of tricuspid regurgitation in patients with prolactinomas chronically treated with cabergoline. J Clin Endocrinol Metab 2008;93(10): 3777–84.

47. Hofland LJ, van der Hoek J, Feelders R, et al. The multi-ligand somatostatin analogue SOM230 inhibits ACTH secretion by cultured human corticotroph adenomas via somatostatin receptor type 5. Eur J Endocrinol 2005;152(4):645–54.

48. Colao A, Petersenn S, Newell-Price J, et al. A 12-month phase 3 study of pasireotide in Cushing's disease. N Engl J Med 2012;366(10):914–24.

49. Lacroix A, Gu F, Gallardo W, et al. Efficacy and safety of once-monthly pasireotide in Cushing's disease: a 12 month clinical trial. Lancet Diabetes Endocrinol 2018;6(1):17–26.

50. Katznelson L. Sustained improvements in plasma ACTH and clinical status in a patient with Nelson's syndrome treated with pasireotide LAR, a multireceptor somatostatin analog. J Clin Endocrinol Metab 2013;98(5):1803–7.

51. Henry RR, Ciaraldi TP, Armstrong D, et al. Hyperglycemia associated with pasireotide: results from a mechanistic study in healthy volunteers. J Clin Endocrinol Metab 2013;98(8):3446–53.

52. Liu JK, Patel J, Eloy JA. The role of temozolomide in the treatment of aggressive pituitary tumors. J Clin Neurosci 2015;22(6):923–9.

53. McCormack AI, Wass JA, Grossman AB. Aggressive pituitary tumours: the role of temozolomide and the assessment of MGMT status. Eur J Clin Invest 2011;41(10):1133–48.

54. Castillo V, Giacomini D, Paez-Pereda M, et al. Retinoic acid as a novel medical therapy for Cushing's disease in dogs. Endocrinology 2006;147(9): 4438–44.

55. Pecori Giraldi F, Ambrogio AG, Andrioli M, et al. Potential role for retinoic acid in patients with Cushing's

disease. J Clin Endocrinol Metab 2012;97(10): 3577–83.

56. Vilar L, Albuquerque JL, Lyra R, et al. The role of iso-tretinoin therapy for Cushing's disease: results of a prospective study. Int J Endocrinol 2016;2016: 8173182.

57. Reincke M, Sbiera S, Hayakawa A, et al. Mutations in the deubiquitinase gene USP8 cause Cushing's disease. Nat Genet 2015;47(1):31–8.

58. Theodoropoulou M, Reincke M, Fassnacht M, et al. Decoding the genetic basis of Cushing's disease: USP8 in the spotlight. Eur J Endocrinol 2015; 173(4):M73–83.

59. Fukuoka H, Cooper O, Ben-Shlomo A, et al. EGFR as a therapeutic target for human, canine, and mouse ACTH-secreting pituitary adenomas. J Clin Invest 2011;121(12):4712–21.

60. Liu NA, Jiang H, Ben-Shlomo A, et al. Targeting zebrafish and murine pituitary corticotroph tumors with a cyclin-dependent kinase (CDK) inhibitor. Proc Natl Acad Sci U S A 2011;108(20):8414–9.

61. Liu NA, Araki T, Cuevas-Ramos D, et al. Cyclin E-mediated human proopiomelanocortin regulation as a therapeutic target for Cushing disease. J Clin Endocrinol Metab 2015;100(7):2557–64.

62. Riebold M, Kozany C, Freiburger L, et al. A C-terminal HSP90 inhibitor restores glucocorticoid sensitivity and relieves a mouse allograft model of Cushing disease. Nat Med 2015;21(3):276–80.

63. Castinetti F, Fassnacht M, Johanssen S, et al. Merits and pitfalls of mifepristone in Cushing's syndrome. Eur J Endocrinol 2009;160(6):1003–10.

64. Fleseriu M, Molitch ME, Gross C, et al. A new therapeutic approach in the medical treatment of Cushing's syndrome: glucocorticoid receptor blockade with mifepristone. Endocr Pract 2013;19(2):313–26.

65. Fleseriu M, Biller BM, Findling JW, et al. Mifepristone, a glucocorticoid receptor antagonist, produces clinical and metabolic benefits in patients with Cushing's syndrome. J Clin Endocrinol Metab 2012;97(6):2039–49.

66. Fleseriu M, Findling JW, Koch CA, et al. Changes in plasma ACTH levels and corticotroph tumor size in patients with Cushing's disease during long-term treatment with the glucocorticoid receptor antagonist mifepristone. J Clin Endocrinol Metab 2014; 99(10):3718–27.

67. Hunt H, Donaldson K, Strem M, et al. Assessment of safety, tolerability, pharmacokinetics, and pharmacological effect of orally administered CORT125134: an adaptive, double-blind, randomized, placebo-controlled phase 1 clinical study. Clin Pharmacol Drug Dev 2018;7(4):408–21.

68. Moraitis A, Agrawal N, Bancos I, et al. Open label phase 2 study to assess safety and efficacy of relacorilant (CORT125134), a selective cortisol modulator, in the treatment of endogenous hypercortisolism. Endocr Pract 2018;24(Supplement 1): 300–1.

69. Barbot M, Albiger N, Ceccato F, et al. Combination therapy for Cushing's disease: effectiveness of two schedules of treatment: should we start with cabergoline or ketoconazole? Pituitary 2014;17(2):109–17.

70. Corcuff JB, Young J, Masquefa-Giraud P, et al. Rapid control of severe neoplastic hypercortisolism with metyrapone and ketoconazole. Eur J Endocrinol 2015;172(4):473–81.

71. Feelders RA, de Bruin C, Pereira AM, et al. Pasireotide alone or with cabergoline and ketoconazole in Cushing's disease. N Engl J Med 2010;362(19): 1846–8.

72. Kamenicky P, Droumaguet C, Salenave S, et al. Mitotane, metyrapone, and ketoconazole combination therapy as an alternative to rescue adrenalectomy for severe ACTH-dependent Cushing's syndrome. J Clin Endocrinol Metab 2011;96(9):2796–804.

The Role of Surgery in the Management of Prolactinomas

Daniel A. Donoho, MD*, Edward R. Laws Jr, MD

KEYWORDS

- Pituitary • Surgery • Transsphenoidal • Prolactinoma • Hyperprolactinemia

KEY POINTS

- Patients never treated with dopamine agonists (DAs) should be considered for surgery if they present with apoplexy or acute onset of neurologic deficits including visual loss, have hyperprolactinemia in the borderline range for stalk effect, or have a cystic prolactinoma.
- Patients previously treated with DAs should be considered for surgery if they are intolerant to DA, as measured by significant subjective symptoms, or fail therapy with at least 1 DA.
- All patients who fail 2 DAs should be considered for surgery.

INTRODUCTION

Pituitary lactotroph adenomas that secrete prolactin (prolactinomas) are the most common functional pituitary adenomas, comprising 40% of all pituitary adenomas.[1] In western countries, prolactinomas have a prevalence of 35 cases per 100,000 population and an annual incidence of 1.6 to 2.2 new cases per 100,000 persons, peaking in women during childbearing years.[2–4] Prolactinomas are also common in patients with multiple endocrine neoplasia, type 1.[5] Consensus guidelines and highly cited review articles describe several common management algorithms for prolactinomas.[1,6] This article will discuss the role of surgery for these patients.

One initial challenge in managing a patient with a potential prolactinoma lies in correctly interpreting the prolactin level. Although a normal prolactin essentially rules out a prolactinoma once appropriately diluted (dilution should be performed for all samples), an elevated prolactin may come from several causes including medication effect, mechanical stimulation of the nipple, macroprolactin, and mass effect from a sellar lesion compressing the pituitary stalk (stalk effect). Because sellar masses can be detected in as many as 10% of patients,[6] it is plausible for a patient with hyperprolactinemia from 1 of the other aforementioned causes to have a coincidental (nonprolactinoma) sellar mass. In 1 series of hyperprolactinemic children and adolescents, more than 50% of patients did not have sellar lesions.[7] Accordingly, the authors have developed an approach that compares the prolactin level to the tumor volume (Burke and colleagues, submitted). Although common guidelines hold that compression of the pituitary stalk from a nonprolactinoma should not raise the prolactin above 150 mcg/L,[6] this cutoff might become as high as 250 mcg/L in macroadenomas or in patients with concomitant stalk effect plus medication effect.[1] Although the sensitivity/specificity of the round figures used in guidelines remains to be assessed, there is growing evidence that these cutoffs should be described in terms of prolactin per cm^3 of tumor[8] rather than absolute prolactin level.

Once a patient is diagnosed with a prolactinoma, the goals of treatment are to prevent

Disclosure Statement: The authors have nothing to disclose.
Department of Neurosurgery, Brigham and Women's Hospital, BTM 4, 60 Fenwood Road, Boston, MA 02115, USA
* Corresponding author.
E-mail address: Daniel.Donoho@med.usc.edu
; @ddonoho (D.A.D.)

Neurosurg Clin N Am 30 (2019) 509–514
https://doi.org/10.1016/j.nec.2019.05.010

neurologic morbidity and to restore endocrine function. Although medical management with a dopamine agonist (DA) is the optimal first-line therapy for many patients, several distinct subsets of patients will require neurosurgical intervention. Surgery should only be performed as part of an integrated management strategy, and each lesion should be considered on a case-by-case basis. Accordingly, the authors consider 2 particular patient groups with hyperprolactinemia and a sellar mass to be potential candidates for surgery.

patients never treated with DA should be considered for surgery if they

Present with apoplexy or acute onset of neurologic deficits including visual loss

Have hyperprolactinemia in the borderline range for stalk effect

Have a cystic prolactinoma

patients previously treated with DA should be considered for surgery if they

Are intolerant to DA, as measured by significant subjective symptoms

Fail therapy with at least 1 DA (all patients who fail 2 DAs should be considered for surgery)

Fig. 1 illustrates the rationale for surgical intervention in our patients who underwent elective surgery for prolactinoma.

SURGERY AS FIRST-LINE THERAPY

Although DAs are the traditional first-line therapy for prolactinomas, a select group of patients should be considered for surgery prior to a trial of DA. These include patients who present with apoplexy or acute onset of neurologic deficits including visual loss, patients who are more likely to have possible stalk effect but for whom diagnostic uncertainty exists, or patients who have a cystic prolactinoma.

Prolactinoma with Apoplexy

Little controversy exists regarding the management of patients with symptomatic pituitary apoplexy, whether from prolactinomas or nonfunctional tumors. Patients with pituitary adenomas and apoplexy should undergo timely neurosurgical intervention. Because the underlying tumor undergoes acute changes in size during the apoplectic event, with resulting neurologic compromise, only treatment modalities that can address that change in size should be considered. Accordingly, surgery is the primary recommended treatment option for symptomatic prolactinoma with apoplexy. The timing of prolactinoma surgery in the setting of apoplexy should be treated with the same urgency as other types of pituitary adenomas.

Prolactinoma with Visual Loss or Other Neurologic Deficits

Patients with neurologic deficits referable to their prolactinoma such as visual field deficits or cranial neuropathies that occur over the subacute period without apoplexy represent an intermediate scenario. Although these patients are among the best candidates for neurosurgical intervention,

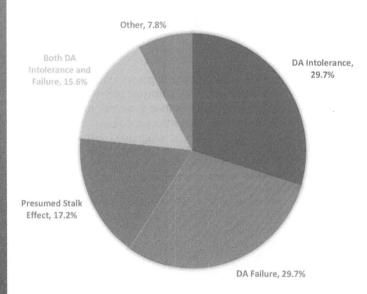

RATIONALE FOR SURGERY FOR PROLACTINOMAS

Other, 7.8%

Both DA Intolerance and Failure, 15.6%

DA Intolerance, 29.7%

Presumed Stalk Effect, 17.2%

DA Failure, 29.7%

Fig. 1. In a single-institution series of 64 patients undergoing elective surgery for immunohistochemically-proven prolactinoma operated by the senior author over 6 years, most patients underwent surgery because of intolerance to adverse effects of DA therapy and/or inability to control prolactin levels at maximal doses of the medication. Only a minority of patients did not attempt a trial of DA therapy prior to surgery. (*Data from* Smith TR, Hulou MM, Huang KT, et al. Current indications for the surgical treatment of prolactinomas. J Clin Neurosci. 2015;22(11):1785–1791.)

carefully selected patients can be managed medically. These patients would include those too sick to safely undergo surgery, patients who elect to avoid surgery, or patients with mild early visual changes. However, it is the authors' common practice that all patients with pituitary adenomas and neurologic deficits referable to the adenoma should undergo neurosurgical consultation. In the authors' practice, almost all of these patients proceed with neurosurgical intervention. **Fig. 2** illustrates the case of a patient with a macroprolactinoma and visual loss who was treated with transsphenoidal surgery.

Cystic Prolactinomas

Patients with cystic prolactinomas are traditionally thought to be less responsive to DA than patients with solid tumors, and current guidelines recommend that these patients undergo surgery first.[1] This may be due to the tumor mass responding less well to the medication or because these patients have more severe symptoms from the mass effect of the hypocellular cyst rather than the hypercellular solid tumor. However, recent studies have questioned whether all patients with cystic prolactinomas but without neurologic deficits should undergo DA therapy just as patients with noncystic prolactinomas do. Faje and colleagues[9] from the Massachusetts General Hospital published a series of 30 patients with cystic prolactinomas: 22 who underwent DA therapy and 8 who had surgery. Although DAs reduced cyst volume in most patients within 2 to 6 months, 7 of 22 patients in the DA first group ultimately required surgery, including 3 patients whose cysts grew or did not shrink. Conversely, all patients undergoing surgery had optic chiasm decompression and reduction in cyst volume. In the hands of an experienced neuroendocrine center, it would be most reasonable to proceed with DA therapy for cystic prolactinomas in patients without chiasmatic compression or neurologic deficits who can be carefully followed.[10] Patients should be counseled that they may not experience an adequate response to therapy and should be vigilant for symptoms of treatment failure. All such patients should be offered the option of transsphenoidal surgery in the hands of an experienced pituitary surgeon.

Patient Preference/Elective Resection

Although patient preference should always be respected, patients who state that they prefer surgery should still have the medical management options and benefits of medical therapy explained to them. If a surgical cure cannot be safely effected, then that should also be explained to patients before scheduling surgery. The authors have found several factors to lead patients in their practice to prefer surgery, including the need for lifelong medication, the preference for definitive management, and the desire to pursue pregnancy in the short term.

One of the main concerns among the authors' patients is the need for lifelong DA therapy. Current guidelines state that DAs should be continued for at least 2 years after normalization of hyperprolactinemia; they subsequently can be tapered in many patients.[11] Although tapering DAs may reduce some adverse effects, including the potential for cardiac valve disease, the need for consistent medication use is onerous for some younger patients for whom prolactinoma is their only medical problem. Although earlier reports used to formulate society guidelines suggested that DAs can discontinued in select

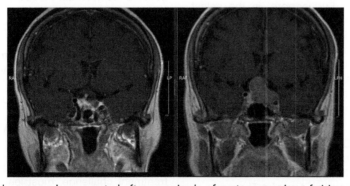

Fig. 2. A 59-year-old woman who presented after an episode of acute worsening of vision and development of adrenal insufficiency. She was found to have a slight left temporal hemianopsia and underwent an MRI. Prolactin was 269. She underwent a transsphenoidal surgery and was discharged on hospital day 2 without complications. Pathology revealed a prolactinoma. Her prolactin subsequent normalized ,and she was tapered off steroids. The left image is taken from her preoperative coronal MRI of the pituitary after gadolinium, and the image on the right is her postoperative coronal MRI after gadolinium.

patients when following a careful algorithm as part of a research protocol, reports of implementation of these guidelines in clinical practice revealed a 60% recurrence rate of hyperprolactinemia requiring medication resumption within 18 months.[12] Accordingly, patients should be counseled that successful medical therapy often requires lifelong DA administration.

A further rationale for surgery is a patient's request for definitive management. The authors have had many patients request that they want to be done with the lesion; how this question is approached depends on local surgical results. If surgery results in hypopituitarism or a residual lesion requiring DA therapy, the authors would not consider surgery a success unless DA therapy had been previously attempted. In the authors' series of primarily DA-resistant and DA-intolerant patients, 67.7% of patients did not require postoperative DAs.[13] When analyzed by indication, 83.9% of DA-intolerant, 64.8% of DA-naïve, and 64.3% of DA-resistant patients were free from the need for postoperative DA. None of these operated patients required permanent hormone replacement for DI or any other endocrinopathy, nor did any have visual worsening.

Short-term fertility outcomes also represent one possible indication for up-front therapy, as the normalization of prolactin and resumption of menstrual cycles can take several months or even 1 to 2 years after beginning DA therapy. However, the evidence of cabergoline's efficacy even in the face of bromocriptine failure should temper enthusiasm for up-front surgery on the basis of return to fertility.[14] In a study by Ono and colleagues, there were no treatment failures, and all women desiring fertility were able to achieve pregnancy after cabergoline. At this time, surgery for fertility restoration should only be undertaken after failure of both DA agents. Furthermore, in the select case of a pregnant mother with a newly diagnosed prolactinoma, medical management should be preferred unless acute severe headaches or visual loss occurs. The risks of general anesthesia and surgery exceed the benefit of surgical resection of a prolactinoma during pregnancy in all other circumstances.

SURGERY AS SECOND-LINE THERAPY FOR PATIENTS PREVIOUSLY TREATED WITH DOPAMINE AGONISTS

Surgery After Dopamine Agonist Therapy – Intolerance

Although DAs are well tolerated in most patients, adverse effects from DA administration are well documented in the literature. These adverse effects often occur in a dose-dependent fashion. This is particularly important when considering that these are medications that are taken for many years (sometimes lifelong). Medication adverse effects were substantial in patients treated with bromocriptine; 78% of patients experienced adverse effects, and more than 5% of patients discontinued the medication, leading to the development of cabergoline approximately 20 years ago.[15] Adverse effects of cabergoline are significantly less frequent compared with bromocriptine, but headache is still common, and rare adverse events such as intratumoral hemorrhage and cerebrospinal fluid leak have been reported consistently since the medication was brought to market.[15] Accordingly, the authors and others have operated on several patients who are intolerant to both DA medications.

Surgery After Dopamine Agonist Therapy – Treatment Failure

Although many patients experience relief of hyperprolactinemia with DA therapy, those who do not demonstrate normalization of prolactin levels should be considered for surgery. Almost half of the authors' surgical cases were operated on after DA treatment failure; 15.6% of their cases exhibited a mixture of treatment failure and adverse effect intolerance, since they did not exhibit normalization of serum prolactin despite reaching maximal dosage levels and were also unable to maintain maximal levels because of medication adverse effects. Surgical results in these patients were favorable, with 60.7% achieving normal prolactin levels after surgery. Other studies indicated a lower rate of response after medical treatment failure compared with patients who had medication intolerance.[16] Because 39.3% of patients did not meet the authors' goal of prolactin normalization, there clearly remains a subset of patients who would benefit from further medical therapy with a different agent. Unfortunately, no other US Food and Drug Administration (FDA)-approved medications are available. Many of these drug-resistant patients require radiation-based treatment for their residual disease.

SURGERY FOR RECURRENT AND AGGRESSIVE PROLACTINOMAS

Recurrent and aggressive prolactinoma is a rare treatment challenge; most lesions are effectively treated using the multimodal paradigm detailed previously. Temozolomide may be of use in these cases, particularly when it is started early in the disease course.[17] Accordingly, all patients with tumors undergoing radiation therapy who have already failed medical and surgical therapy should be closely monitored, and chemotherapy should be considered.

Prolactinomas rarely progress to pituitary carcinoma. Carcinomas, diagnosed on the basis of their metastases, often have extremely elevated MIB-1 and p53 expression and portend a poor prognosis.[18,19] Short-term treatment success can occur if the metastases can be resected en bloc.[20] However, the long-term outlook for these patients remains unclear, and late metastases can still occur with fatal results.

SUMMARY

Prolactinomas represent a common, but complex neuroendocrine challenge. Prolactinoma patients should be cared for at a high-volume neuroendocrine center that includes neuroendocrinologists, neurosurgeons, neuroradiologists, and other staff with experience in managing pituitary disease. If these patients are managed outside of high-volume centers, they should be urgently referred if there is any indication that the prolactin is not under control and normalizing, the tumor is growing, or if the patient has any change in neurologic function.

Prolactinomas are most commonly managed medically using DA therapy. Typically, the best care for these patients will occur at high-volume pituitary neuroendocrine centers. All patients who have neurologic symptoms referable to the lesion, who desire more information about surgery, or who are at risk for treatment failure should meet with a neurosurgeon experienced in transsphenoidal surgery. In select patients, including those with acute visual loss, intolerance to medical therapy, or treatment failures, surgical intervention should be strongly considered. In the era of endoscopic endonasal surgery, surgical remission rates are high in carefully selected patients, and transsphenoidal surgery should be considered in the scenarios that have been outlined in this article. The authors are hopeful that further progress in surgical adjuncts may help make transsphenoidal surgery even more efficacious in the future.

REFERENCES

1. Casanueva FF, Molitch ME, Schlechte JA, et al. Guidelines of the Pituitary Society for the diagnosis and management of prolactinomas. Clin Endocrinol (Oxf) 2006;65(2):265–73.

2. Gruppetta M, Mercieca C, Vassallo J. Prevalence and incidence of pituitary adenomas: a population based study in Malta. Pituitary 2013;16(4):545–53.

3. Tjornstrand A, Gunnarsson K, Evert M, et al. The incidence rate of pituitary adenomas in western Sweden for the period 2001-2011. Eur J Endocrinol 2014;171(4):519–26.

4. Raappana A, Koivukangas J, Ebeling T, et al. Incidence of pituitary adenomas in northern Finland in 1992-2007. J Clin Endocrinol Metab 2010;95(9): 4268–75.

5. de Laat JM, Dekkers OM, Pieterman CR, et al. Long-term natural course of pituitary tumors in patients with MEN1: results from the DutchMEN1 Study Group (DMSG). J Clin Endocrinol Metab 2015; 100(9):3288–96.

6. Klibanski A. Clinical practice. Prolactinomas. N Engl J Med 2010;362(13):1219–26.

7. Eren E, Torel Ergur A, Isguven SP, et al. Clinical and laboratory characteristics of hyperprolactinemia in children and adolescents: national survey. J Clin Res Pediatr Endocrinol 2019;11(2):149–56.

8. Huang Y, Ding C, Zhang F, et al. Role of prolactin/adenoma maximum diameter and prolactin/adenoma volume in the differential diagnosis of prolactinomas and other types of pituitary adenomas. Oncol Lett 2018;15(2):2010–6.

9. Faje A, Chunharojrith P, Nency J, et al. Dopamine agonists can reduce cystic prolactinomas. J Clin Endocrinol Metab 2016;101(10):3709–15.

10. Nakhleh A, Shehadeh N, Hochberg I, et al. Management of cystic prolactinomas: a review. Pituitary 2018;21(4):425–30.

11. Paepegaey AC, Salenave S, Kamenicky P, et al. Cabergoline tapering is almost always successful in patients with macroprolactinomas. J Endocr Soc 2017;1(3):221–30.

12. Kharlip J, Salvatori R, Yenokyan G, et al. Recurrence of hyperprolactinemia after withdrawal of long-term cabergoline therapy. J Clin Endocrinol Metab 2009;94(7):2428–36.

13. Smith TR, Hulou MM, Huang KT, et al. Current indications for the surgical treatment of prolactinomas. J Clin Neurosci 2015;22(11): 1785–91.

14. Ono M, Miki N, Amano K, et al. Individualized high-dose cabergoline therapy for hyperprolactinemic infertility in women with micro- and macroprolactinomas. J Clin Endocrinol Metab 2010;95(6): 2672–9.

15. Biller BM, Molitch ME, Vance ML, et al. Treatment of prolactin-secreting macroadenomas with the once-weekly dopamine agonist cabergoline. J Clin Endocrinol Metab 1996;81(6):2338–43.

16. Hamilton DK, Vance ML, Boulos PT, et al. Surgical outcomes in hyporesponsive prolactinomas: analysis of patients with resistance or intolerance to dopamine agonists. Pituitary 2005; 8(1):53–60.

17. Barkhoudarian G, Palejwala SK, Ogunbameru R, et al. Early recognition and initiation of temozolomide chemotherapy for refractory, invasive pituitary macroprolactinoma with long-term sustained remission. World Neurosurg 2018;118:118–24.

18. Hansen TM, Batra S, Lim M, et al. Invasive adenoma and pituitary carcinoma: a SEER database analysis. Neurosurg Rev 2014;37(2):279–85 [discussion: 285–6].

19. Phillips J, East HE, French SE, et al. What causes a prolactinoma to be aggressive or to become a pituitary carcinoma? Hormones (Athens) 2012;11(4): 477–82.

20. Seltzer J, Carmichael JD, Commins D, et al. Prolactin-secreting pituitary carcinoma with dural metastasis: diagnosis, treatment, and future directions. World Neurosurg 2016;91:676. e23-8.

Sodium Perturbations After Pituitary Surgery

Kevin C.J. Yuen, MD, FRCP (UK)[a],*, Adnan Ajmal, MD[b], Ricardo Correa, MD, EdD[c], Andrew S. Little, MD[d]

KEYWORDS

- Pituitary surgery • Hypernatremia • Hyponatremia • Diabetes Insipidus • SIADH
- Transsphenoidal surgery

KEY POINTS

- Sodium perturbations are a common complication after pituitary surgery, with hyponatremia being the most frequent complication and the reason for hospital readmission.
- Postoperative assessments should be tailored to the early (immediately after surgery through the following first few weeks) and late postoperative periods (after 6 weeks postoperatively to months).
- Monitoring sodium perturbations due to deficiency or excess antidiuretic hormone manifesting as diabetes insipidus or SIADH, respectively, is recommended.
- Cerebral salt wasting is a rare phenomenon after pituitary surgery, and the diagnosis and management can be challenging especially when it coexists with SIADH.
- Providing patient counseling and close postoperative follow-up is important to effectively manage diabetes insipidus and reduce hospital readmissions due to sodium perturbations.

INTRODUCTION

Pituitary adenomas are the third most common intracranial tumor, accounting for 10% to 15% of all diagnosed intracranial neoplasms, and are frequently treated with transsphenoidal surgery (TSS).[1] Although the rates of morbidity and mortality are reportedly low after TSS at high-volume neurosurgical centers,[2,3] changes in postoperative anterior and posterior pituitary function, particularly sodium perturbations due to changes in antidiuretic hormone (ADH) secretion, remains one of the most frequent postoperative complications and reasons for hospital readmissions.[4–8] The predisposition to develop sodium perturbations are multifactorial, and the following factors have been reported to adversely affect the rates of this complication: younger age, male gender, greater tumor volume, preoperative pituitary function, the number of previous pituitary surgeries, first postoperative sodium that exceeds 145 mmol/L, the extent of the resection (gross vs subtotal resection), surgery for microadenomas (possibly secondary to stalk manipulation

Disclosure: The authors have nothing to disclose.
[a] Department of Neuroendocrinology, Barrow Pituitary Center, Barrow Neurological Institute, St. Joseph's Hospital and Medical Center, University of Arizona College of Medicine and Creighton School of Medicine, 124 W Thomas Road, Suite 300, Phoenix, AZ 85013, USA; [b] Department of Internal Medicine and Endocrinology, St. Joseph's Hospital and Medical Center, Creighton University School of Medicine, 500 W Thomas Road, Suite 900B Phoenix, AZ 85013, USA; [c] Department of Medicine, Division of Endocrinology, Diabetes and Metabolism, Phoenix Veterans Administration Medical Center, University of Arizona College of Medicine, Creighton School of Medicine and Mayo School of Medicine, 650 E Indian School Road, Building 21, Suite 117, Phoenix, AZ 85014, USA; [d] Department of Neurosurgery, Barrow Pituitary Center, Barrow Neurological Institute, St. Joseph's Hospital and Medical Center, University of Arizona College of Medicine, 300 W Thomas Road, Phoenix, AZ 85013, USA
* Corresponding author.
E-mail address: kevin.yuen@dignityhealth.org

and exploration), intrasellar expansion of the tumor, intraoperative cerebrospinal fluid (CSF) leak, nonpituitary sellar lesions such as craniopharyngiomas, and tumor type (Cushing disease is the most common type).[4,5,9–11] Therefore, concerted efforts should be made to preidentify risk factors for developing postoperative sodium perturbations to minimize the risk of hospital readmissions. Postoperative assessments should be specifically tailored to the early (immediately after surgery through the following first few weeks) and late postoperative periods (after 6 weeks postoperatively to months). Despite this pervasive problem, consensus guidelines for optimal postoperative management are still scarce, although recent studies have demonstrated the usefulness of adhering to fluid restrictions ranging from less than 1.0[12] to 1.5 L[13] per day to reduce the rate of hospital readmissions for delayed hyponatremia after TSS.

Therefore, the aim of this article is to discuss the diagnostic and therapeutic challenges of managing postoperative sodium perturbations, and describe strategies for assessment and monitoring of the patient after pituitary surgery to decrease hospitalization readmission rates. These challenges apply for patients who have undergone pituitary surgery via the transsphenoidal and transcranial route.

PHYSIOLOGY OF WATER AND SODIUM HOMEOSTASIS

Water metabolism is primarily controlled by ADH, which is synthesized in the neurons of the supraoptic and paraventricular nuclei of the hypothalamus and is stored in the posterior pituitary gland. Plasma osmolality (ratio of solutes to water in the blood plasma) is the principal stimulus for ADH secretion, whereas blood pressure and blood volume contribute to a lesser extent.[14] Osmoreceptors in the hypothalamus are the major contributor of water regulation, as they are sensitive to changes in plasma osmolality. In addition, baroreceptors located in the carotid arteries and aortic arch also affect ADH secretion in response to decreases in blood volume or arterial pressure. The resulting urinary concentration and renal water conservation is an appropriate physiologic response to the volume depletion.[15]

When secreted, ADH binds to the V2 receptors in the renal collecting ducts, activating a cyclic AMP-mediated signal transduction pathway that stimulates insertion of aquaporin-2 water channels into the apical membrane of the collecting duct epithelial cells. These water channels increase water permeability that facilitates passive renal water reabsorption, which consequently alters plasma sodium levels.[15] In addition, the thirst mechanism also plays an important role in maintaining water and sodium homeostasis. If plasma osmolality increases, the thirst center in the cerebral cortex is stimulated to promote increased water intake. Mild to moderate changes in plasma sodium levels can cause changes in endogenous ADH secretion. When the plasma sodium level rises above 145 mmol/L, plasma osmolality increases, which subsequently increases ADH secretion. Conversely, when the plasma sodium level decreases to less than 135 mmol/L, plasma osmolality decreases, which consequently decreases ADH secretion.

HYPERNATREMIA AFTER PITUITARY SURGERY

Postoperative hypernatremia is typically caused by the development of diabetes insipidus (DI), which tends to occur during the acute phase after pituitary surgery,[16] manifesting as hypotonic polyuria, with urine volumes ranging from 3.5 to 16.8 L per day.[17] Surgical manipulation of pituitary stalk and posterior pituitary gland, excision of neurohypophysis, and hemi-hypophysectomy are possible mechanisms.[18] Overall incidence is reported to be 1.6% to 45% for transient DI and 0.3% to 10% for persistent DI after pituitary surgery.[19] Several studies have shown that endoscopic TSS has a lower incidence of postoperative DI compared with the microscopic approach (11% to 15% in endoscopic vs 22% to 28% in microscopic groups),[20,21] whereas others have not shown any differences.[22,23] However, in a recent large multicenter study comparing endoscopic versus microscopic TSS, postoperative DI was also reported to be less common in the endoscopic group, although the rates were lower compared with previous studies (2.4% in endoscopic vs 8.9% in microscopic groups).[24] In most cases, DI manifests shortly after pituitary surgery (1–3 days postoperatively), although delayed DI is also reported in patients with Rathke's cleft cyst.[25] In such patients, the mechanism of delayed DI is not well understood, but it is thought to be related to the release of cyst contents causing inflammation near the neurohypophysis.[26] Conversely, hypernatremia can rapidly ensue in the presence of thirst abnormalities such as adipsia or hypodipsia from hypothalamic osmoreceptor damage, or if the patient is unconscious or cognitively impaired.

The diagnosis of postoperative DI can be challenging owing to multiple confounding factors, such as the administration of anesthesia, and medications such as diuretics and perioperative intravenous (IV) fluid infusions. Furthermore, the diagnostic criteria of postoperative DI is not uniform, with most studies adopting several of the following criteria to arrive at the diagnosis, including polyuria greater than 300 mL/h for 2 consecutive hours or greater than 3.0 L per day, urine specific gravity less than 1.005, plasma sodium greater than 140 to 145 mmol/L, plasma osmolality greater than 300 mmol/L, and urine osmolality less than 200 to 300 mOsm/kg with blood glucose levels less than 180 mg/dL.[11,17,19] It is noteworthy that other causes of polyuria such as postoperative water diuresis, diabetes mellitus, and glucocorticoid-induced hyperglycemia causing osmotic diuresis must be excluded.[27] In addition, hypotonic polyuria can occur when there is rapid fluid loss from extravascular soft tissues in patients with acromegaly after successful pituitary surgery, which may be misdiagnosed as DI.[18]

Several studies have assessed the perioperative risk factors for the development of DI in an effort to identify patients earlier. Greater tumor volume, first postoperative plasma sodium that exceeds 145 mmol/L, intraoperative CSF leak, functional corticotroph tumors, Rathke's cleft cyst, and craniopharyngioma are associated with an increased risk of early postoperative DI after pituitary surgery,[10,11,19,28,29] whereas younger age, larger tumor size, gross total resection, and reoperation due to possible injury to the neurohypophysis and/or stalk traction were associated with persistent DI.[18,19] By contrast, preoperative and postoperative glucocorticoid use in short-term and long-term periods do not confer an increased risk for persistent DI,[19] whereas diuretic use and chronic hyperglycemia are not associated with an increased risk of DI but may cause hypertonic polyuria.[10]

HYPONATREMIA AFTER PITUITARY SURGERY

Postoperative hyponatremia is frequently caused by syndrome of inappropriate ADH (SIADH), which could be isolated or part of a biphasic[30] or triphasic response,[9,31,32] and rarely by cerebral salt wasting (CSW) syndrome.[33] However, differentiation between SIADH and CSW is often challenging. The main clinical difference between the 2 conditions is the volume status of the patient. CSW syndrome is characterized by increased natriuresis (urine sodium >100 mmol/L), diuresis, and a subsequent volume depletion state, whereas the clinical manifestations of SIADH include inappropriate free water retention, mild

natriuresis, and a euvolemic state.[34] Delayed hyponatremia tends to present between 4 to 12 days with a peak incidence of 7 to 8 days postoperatively.[4] Previous studies have reported this incidence to range between 1.8% and 35%,[35] although an earlier study by Sane and colleagues[36] reported the incidence to be as high as 61%.

The pathophysiology of postoperative hyponatremia is not well understood, but is thought to be due to the changes in ADH release from ADH-producing neurons in the surgically manipulated posterior pituitary cells.[37,38] Hence, when assessing a postsurgical patient, it is imperative to exclude the presence of concurrent hypothyroidism and adrenal insufficiency (AI),[39] as thyroid hormone and cortisol may inhibit ADH release.[40,41] Risk factors for developing postoperative hyponatremia include the tumor size, patient age, preoperative pituitary function, and whether the patient had undergone prior pituitary surgeries.[42]

The clinical features of postoperative hyponatremia can range from being asymptomatic to nonspecific, for example, headache, nausea, vomiting, lethargy, restlessness, disorientation, and depressed reflexes, and following the rapid decline of plasma sodium levels, convulsions, stupor, and coma.[32,43] In a study by Sata and colleagues,[35] 22% of the patients who developed symptomatic hyponatremia were patients with macroadenomas, and that plasma sodium levels less than 105 mmol/L was associated with more than 50% mortality rate. The excess mortality rate is related to central pontine and extrapontine myelinolysis due to rapid changes of the plasma sodium levels.[43] Therefore, it is important to cautiously correct the plasma sodium levels to achieve normonatremia so as not exceed 10 to 12 mmol/L changes during the first 24 hours, and 18 mmol/L over the next 48 hours.[44]

THE "TRIPHASIC RESPONSE" OF POSTOPERATIVE DIABETES INSIPIDUS

The course of postoperative DI may be transient, persistent, or triphasic. The triphasic response is observed in 3.4% of patients after TSS (**Fig. 1**), whereas the first 2 phases occur in only 1.1% of patients.[30] In the triphasic response, a polyuric phase of DI is followed by an oliguric phase of SIADH, and then by a third and final phase of persistent DI.[45] The initial transient phase of DI occurs within postoperative days 1 and 3 after TSS that typically lasts for 5 to 7 days. This phase is initiated following a partial or complete pituitary

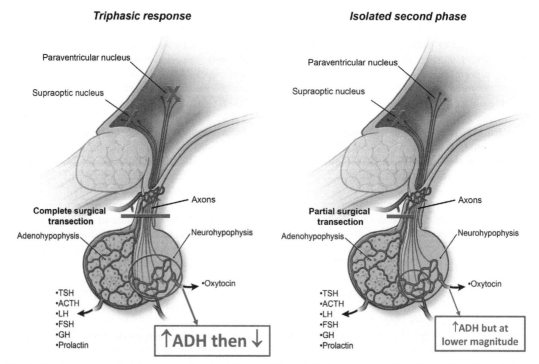

Fig. 1. Mechanisms underlying the pathophysiology of the triphasic response of postoperative DI and the isolated second phase. X, depletion of ADH stores; ↑, increased; ↓, decreased. (Used with permission from Barrow Neurological Institute.)

stalk transection with resultant edema and/or axonal shock from disruption of the vascular supply to the pituitary stalk, which in turn severs the connections between the ADH neuronal cell bodies in the hypothalamus and the nerve terminals in the posterior pituitary gland, thus decreasing stimulated endogenous ADH secretion. Transient DI then resolves when there is recovery of ADH-secreting neurons.[46] If there is no recovery, the second phase will ensue, caused by the uncontrolled release of ADH from either degenerating posterior pituitary tissue or from the remaining magnocellular neurons, whose axons have been damaged, that can last from 2 to 14 days with a peak at days 7 to 8 postoperatively. During this phase, urine output decreases and, consequently, urine becomes concentrated. Partial damage to some of the axons in the posterior pituitary may result in isolated second phase SIADH with milder symptoms of hyponatremia.[46] After all of the ADP stored in the posterior pituitary gland has been released, the third and final phase occurs when DI reappears due to the depletion of ADH stores from the retrograde degeneration of hypothalamic ADH-secreting neuronal cell bodies.[47,48]

In some patients, an isolated second phase has been observed following partial transection of the pituitary stalk (see **Fig. 1**). Although

maximum ADH secretory response is diminished as a result of the stalk injury, DI will not be apparent if the injury leaves intact some nerve fibers connecting the ADH neuronal cell bodies in the hypothalamus to the nerve terminals in the posterior pituitary gland. This is followed in several days by the second phase of SIADH, which is caused by the uncontrolled release of ADH from the degenerating nerve terminals of the posterior pituitary gland that have been severed. Because a smaller portion of the posterior pituitary is denervated, the magnitude of ADH released as the pituitary degenerates is smaller and of shorter duration than with a complete triphasic response.[46] After all of the ADH stored in the damaged part of the posterior pituitary gland has been released, the second phase ceases, but clinical DI will not be apparent if there is still functional ADH neuronal cell bodies in the hypothalamus that continue to secrete stimulated ADH, albeit at a lower magnitude.[46]

CEREBRAL SALT WASTING

CSW is a rare condition, which is predominantly associated with subarachnoid hemorrhage,[49,50] but can also rarely occur after pituitary surgery.[33,51] This condition is characterized by polyuria, hypovolemia, and natriuresis, leading to hyponatremia. The exact mechanism underlying CSW is unclear but may involve increased levels of circulating natriuretic peptides, such as atrial natriuretic peptide or brain natriuretic peptide, and decreased sympathetic stimulation to the kidney. These factors increase urinary sodium excretion and diminish effective arterial blood volume, which increases baroreceptor release of ADH to maintain intravascular volume.[52] Concurrently, a decreased sympathetic drive decreases renin and aldosterone levels, further reducing sodium retention.[53] Among patients with central nervous system disease, CSW is a much less common cause of hyponatremia than SIADH.[54,55]

Both CSW and SIADH can coexist in patients with hyponatremia after pituitary surgery,[51] and differentiating these 2 conditions is challenging but important for appropriate treatment implementation. Free water and salt supplementation are the primary therapies for CSW, and conversely, fluid restriction is required for SIADH. CSW and SIADH both present with low plasma osmolality and inappropriately high urine osmolality, with natriuresis (urinary sodium losses >40 mmol/L). However, although the urinary sodium excretion is markedly higher than sodium intake in CSW, it generally equals the sodium intake in SIADH. Therefore, there is a negative net sodium balance in CSW with polyuria and consequent hypovolemia, whereas, in SIADH, patients are generally euvolemic.[52,53] **Table 1** summarizes the main differences in clinical and biochemical parameters between these 2 conditions.

For patients with CSW, early appropriate fluid therapy with isotonic or hypertonic fluids and oral salt supplementation should be initiated. Mineralocorticoid administration (fludrocortisone) can also be used at doses of 0.025 to 1 mg/d to promote sodium retention.[56,57] Once the underlying cause is corrected, CSW is usually a transient condition that resolves within 3 to 4 weeks. In patients in whom CSW and DI coexist,[51] sodium loss due to CSW in itself contributes to the polyuria, and higher desmopressin doses should be avoided as this increases renal free water reabsorption and may cause worsening of the hyponatremia. Treatment consists of careful sodium and fluid replacement, titrated against losses, and cautious continuation of desmopressin, with close monitoring of electrolytes and plasma osmolality.

POSTOPERATIVE ASSESSMENT AND MANAGEMENT

After pituitary surgery, DI is generally more frequently encountered in the early postoperative

Table 1
Summary of differences in clinical and biochemical parameters between cerebral salt wasting versus syndrome of inappropriate antidiuretic hormone

	CSW	SIADH
Body weight	Same or ↓	↑
Extracellular volume	↓	↑
Signs or symptoms of dehydration	Present	Absent
Central venous pressure	↓	Same or ↑
Plasma sodium	↓	↓
Urine sodium	↑	↑
Net sodium loss	↑	Normal
Urine output	↑	↓
Plasma osmolality	↓	↓
Urine osmolality	↑	↑
Plasma urea	Normal or ↑	↓
Plasma ADH	↓	↑
Hematocrit	Normal or ↑	↓
Plasma aldosterone	↓	Normal or ↑
Plasma renin	Normal, ↑ or ↓	↓
Treatment	Salt supplementation and fluid replacement	Fluid restriction

Abbreviations: ↑, increased; ↓, decreased.

period than SIADH,[9] although SIADH may be more common if the surgery is performed endoscopically, which may be because of the expertise of the neurosurgeon in better preserving the posterior pituitary gland.[24] Although its overall incidence is low when the surgery is performed by an experienced neurosurgeon, DI can be challenging to treat, may lengthen the hospital stay, and if not well managed can be fatal. Several studies have examined the incidence of DI after TSS for pituitary adenomas. In some earlier studies, dilute polyuria and polydipsia on the first postoperative day was reported in 34% of 1571 patients with pituitary adenomas,[30] and in 18.3% of 881 patients with a variety of sellar lesions.[28] In these studies, 24%[30] and 12.4%[28] of patients, respectively, required transient therapy with desmopressin. Persistent DI after TSS is fortunately rare and much less common than transient DI. In

1 study, persistent DI was reported at 3 months in 0.9% and at 1 year in 0.25% of patients[30]; in other studies, 2%[28] had persistent DI and 1.4%[18] had persistent DI requiring desmopressin therapy.

Because DI presents clinically with large volumes of dilute urine, plasma osmolality increases, and patients with an intact thirst mechanism may experience an increase in thirst, particularly craving cold liquids. If fluid intake is not increased to compensate for the polyuria, plasma osmolality and sodium will continue to increase. We recommend that all patients who have undergone pituitary surgery require continuous 24-hour close monitoring of fluid intake and urine output, assessment of urinary specific gravity, and daily or twice daily (if DI develops) electrolyte monitoring (**Box 1**). In the absence of hyperglycemia, a low urine specific gravity (<1.005) combined with a high urine volume of greater than 300 mL/h for 2 consecutive hours is highly suggestive of DI. We also recommend close monitoring of plasma and urine osmolality, and electrolytes. Urine output alone cannot be used to diagnose DI because other situations in the postoperative period can increase urine output. The most common is the excretion of fluids administered during the surgical procedure, but this should not be accompanied by hypernatremia or excess thirst.[58] One underrated diagnostic tool at a clinician's disposal is to visually assess the color of the patient's urine. Patients with DI typically excrete clear dilute urine, whereas patients with postoperative diuresis will often excrete yellow-colored urine.

Various strategies are used to treat DI, once confirmed, including drinking to thirst without desmopressin, intermittent as required desmopressin use, and/or scheduled desmopressin use as an outpatient on hospital discharge.[59] If the patient is awake and alert with an intact thirst mechanism, most cases of early postoperative DI can be managed with ad libitum oral intake of fluids and close monitoring.[60] Treatment with desmopressin is required if urine output is excessive (especially at night preventing sleep), if urine output significantly exceeds fluid intake, or if hypernatremia is developing[28] (see **Box 1**). It is important to keep in mind that, during the first 2 weeks postoperatively, desmopressin should be used cautiously because its unrestricted use without a treatment plan can cause hyponatremia due to overtreatment in 40% of the patients.[17] However, if DI worsens and hypernatremia ensues (sodium levels >145 mmol/L), desmopressin can be administered initially on an "as required basis" or at bedtime to reduce nocturia and help with sleep.[18] Patients with an impaired thirst mechanism are clearly more challenging to manage, with higher risks of dehydration and hypernatremia that are associated with increased morbidity and mortality. In these patients, DI needs to be promptly recognized. We recommend obligate urine output monitoring with a fixed amount of desmopressin and a flexible amount of water intake to maintain euvolemia and normal osmolality. This task requires daily weighing, monitoring of urine output, and frequent measuring of plasma sodium and osmolality.[61] If the triphasic response occurs because DI is in most cases transient, regular desmopressin administration can be considered if polyuria persists beyond 48 hours. It is important to continue monitoring plasma sodium levels closely after starting desmopressin and to advise patients and caregivers about the potential risk of the triphasic response, and the need for urgent blood draws to check for plasma sodium levels should the patient develop symptoms suggestive of hyponatremia. Withdrawal of desmopressin before discharge from hospital is useful in identifying those who demonstrate spontaneous return of endogenous ADH secretion. The dose of desmopressin required is proportional to the degree of ADH deficiency. In those with partial DI, a nocturnal oral dose of 0.1 mg may suffice, whereas

---

Box 1
Clinical assessments for sodium perturbations after pituitary surgery

Diabetes insipidus

- Continuous strict monitoring of urine output and fluid intake
- Urine specific gravity measurements
- Measurement of electrolytes at days 5 to 7 postoperatively
- Monitoring of thirst and volume status
- In the absence of hyperglycemia, polyuria (>300 mL/h for 2 consecutive h or 3 L per day), urine specific gravity <1.005, and urine osmolality <250 mOsm/kg is usually due to DI
- Measurement of electrolytes emergently in any unwell patient (headache, nausea, vomiting, dehydration, mental status changes, or seizures)

SIADH

- Home assessments of fluid intake and urine output after discharge in patients on fluid restriction of 1 L per day
- Measurement of electrolytes at days 5 to 7 and at 12 to 14 postoperatively
- Measurement of electrolytes emergently in any unwell patient (headache, nausea, vomiting, mental status changes, or seizures)

those with more severe disease may require higher doses up to 0.2 mg 2 to 3 times per day.

After postoperative days 4 to 7, patients with DI can be instructed to periodically hold their desmopressin for a few hours to assess if polyuria and polydipsia are still present,[62] and if not, desmopressin may be discontinued. The patient will also need to be counseled to continue to monitor his/her fluid intake and urine output at home, and if symptoms of polyuria and/or polydipsia return, reinitiation of desmopressin either "as required" or as scheduled dosing with low initial doses can be considered with periodic follow-up with electrolyte checks performed.

In patients without DI, there is now increasing evidence that supports the implementation of fluid restriction on hospital discharge after pituitary surgery to preemptively decrease the risk of delayed hyponatremia from SIADH. Takeuchi and colleagues,[63] Matsuyama and colleagues,[64] Burke and colleagues,[12] and Deaver and colleagues[13] showed that implementing fluid restrictions of 2.5 L per day for the first 10 postoperative days, 1.6 to 1.8 L per day based on postoperative day 6 sodium levels, 1.0 L per day for the first 7 postoperative days, and 1.5 L per day for the first 14 postoperative days, respectively, consistently decreased hospital readmission rates for hyponatremia. At our institution, we have instituted a protocol of prophylactic fluid restriction in selected patients, and have noted a marked decrease in unplanned readmission rates (see details below). One potential concern, however, about prophylactic fluid restriction is the unintended consequence of increasing the rate of hypernatremia; however, in our experience, we have not observed such readmissions for hypernatremia. Interestingly, Lockett and colleagues[65] recently demonstrated the effectiveness and safety of urea treatment in patients with SIADH and moderate to profound hyponatremia who are unable to undergo or have failed fluid restriction. Nevertheless, large prospective studies are still needed to validate this approach in patients after pituitary surgery, especially to those with specific pituitary pathologies, such as craniopharyngiomas without DI and Cushing disease.

It is critical to establish the cause of hyponatremia because treatment regimens vary. Hypothyroidism and AI should be assessed, and if confirmed, should be treated with appropriate hormone replacement. Isolated hyponatremia without an earlier phase of DI after TSS is typically due to SIADH if hypothyroidism and AI have been excluded, and has been reported in 25%[66] to 23%[67] of patients. A systematic review of 2974 patients from 10 case series found that the frequency of delayed hyponatremia ranged from 3.6% to 19.8%,[5] whereas some studies have shown that the peak time of hyponatremia occurrences is on postoperative day 7 when patients are not monitoring themselves at home.[8,68] In a series of 1571 patients who underwent pituitary surgery, 2.7% developed hyponatremia on postoperative day 1, 1.7% on day 3, and 5% on day 7.[30] This series reported a biphasic pattern (DI followed by SIADH) in 3.4% and triphasic pattern (DI, SIADH, then DI again) in 1.1% of the cohort,[30] whereas hyponatremia was symptomatic in 2.1%.[30] The rate of hyponatremia increased to 40% among patients who had received desmopressin transiently for polyuria, which is much higher than the overall rate of hyponatremia in 24% of the cohort.[30] In another study of 241 patients, 23% developed sodium levels less than 135 mmol/L,[67] whereas the incidence of symptomatic hyponatremia was 5%.[67]

At our institution, which is in a desert climate, we routinely implement a protocol of fluid restriction in selected patients of 1.5 L per day for the first 10 postoperative days, and obtain an electrolyte panel at days 5 to 7 (see **Box 1**). Eligible patients included those with pituitary adenomas and Rathke's cleft cyst without evidence of DI, and we excluded pregnant patients and patients taking loop diuretics. Patients with transient DI, who are at increased risk for SIADH, are instructed to monitor their fluid intake and urine output at home, and to notify our office promptly if urine output falls or increases significantly or if they develop profound thirst. We instruct our patients to monitor themselves for symptoms of hyponatremia, such as headache, dizziness, nausea, vomiting, and altered mental status. However, there is a clear overlap with these symptoms and those of AI. Hence, we also routinely check postoperative morning plasma cortisol levels and offer glucocorticoid supplementation if there is suspicion for AI. If patients have signs or symptoms of SIADH, we recommend emergent checks of plasma sodium levels. If mild hyponatremia (sodium levels 130–135 mmol/L) is present, the patient could continue on their fluid restriction of 1.5 L per day, consume liberal salt intake in their diet, and undergo daily electrolyte panel checks until plasma sodium levels show an upward trend of improvement. If moderate to significant hyponatremia is present (sodium levels <130 mmol/L), we recommend hospitalizing the patient. While in hospital, close monitoring of fluid balance is commenced, and treatment is initiated emergently starting with fluid restriction (800–1000 mL per day depending on the severity of hyponatremia), followed by IV hypertonic saline infusion if fluid restriction fails, and ADH antagonist receptor (V-2 receptors) (eg, oral tolvaptan or intravenous conivaptan) therapy if both fluid restriction and IV hypertonic saline fails.[33,69–71]

SUMMARY

The management of sodium perturbations after pituitary surgery remains challenging for clinicians, and, in the early postoperative period, requires regular patient counseling, consideration of desmopressin therapy for patients with compensated and uncompensated DI, fluid restriction for patients without DI, postoperative assessment for possible hypothyroidism and AI, and a low threshold for performing electrolyte panel checks in any unwell patient after hospital discharge. Ideally, these patients should be managed at specialist centers for pituitary disorders by designated multidisciplinary teams with access to intensive care facilities. In the late postoperative phase, providing regular patient counseling and close postoperative follow-up remains essential to effectively manage DI and reduce hospital readmissions due to sodium perturbations. Further research is needed to identify biochemical and molecular markers that could help the clinician to reliably predict changes in postoperative sodium levels to reduce the risk of hospital readmissions of these patients.

REFERENCES

1. Villwock JA, Villwock M, Deshaies E, et al. Significant increases of pituitary tumors and resections from 1993 to 2011. Int Forum Allergy Rhinol 2014;4: 767–70.
2. Barker FG 2nd, Klibanski A, Swearingen B. Transsphenoidal surgery for pituitary tumors in the United States, 1996-2000: mortality, morbidity, and the effects of hospital and surgeon volume. J Clin Endocrinol Metab 2003;88:4709–19.
3. Solari D, Zenga F, Angileri FF, et al. A survey on pituitary surgery in Italy. World Neurosurg 2018;123: e440–9.
4. Bohl MA, Ahmad S, Jahnke H, et al. Delayed hyponatremia is the most common cause of 30-day unplanned readmission after transsphenoidal surgery for pituitary tumors. Neurosurgery 2016;78: 84–90.
5. Cote DJ, Alzarea A, Acosta MA, et al. Predictors and rates of delayed symptomatic hyponatremia after transsphenoidal surgery: a systematic review [corrected]. World Neurosurg 2016;88:1–6.
6. Cote DJ, Dasenbrock HH, Muskens IS, et al. Readmission and other adverse events after transsphenoidal surgery: prevalence, timing, and predictive factors. J Am Coll Surg 2017;224:971–9.
7. Hendricks BL, Shikary TA, Zimmer LA. Causes for 30-day readmission following transsphenoidal surgery. Otolaryngol Head Neck Surg 2016;154: 359–65.
8. Krogh J, Kistorp CN, Jafar-Mohammadi B, et al. Transsphenoidal surgery for pituitary tumours: frequency and predictors of delayed hyponatraemia and their relationship to early readmission. Eur J Endocrinol 2018;178:247–53.
9. Kiran Z, Sheikh A, Momin SN, et al. Sodium and water imbalance after sellar, suprasellar, and parasellar surgery. Endocr Pract 2017;23:309–17.
10. Nayak P, Montaser AS, Hu J, et al. Predictors of postoperative diabetes insipidus following endoscopic resection of pituitary adenomas. J Endocr Soc 2018;2:1010–9.
11. Schreckinger M, Walker B, Knepper J, et al. Postoperative diabetes insipidus after endoscopic transsphenoidal surgery. Pituitary 2013;16:445–51.
12. Burke WT, Cote DJ, Iuliano SI, et al. A practical method for prevention of readmission for symptomatic hyponatremia following transsphenoidal surgery. Pituitary 2018;21:25–31.
13. Deaver KE, Catel CP, Lillehei KO, et al. Strategies to reduce readmissions for hyponatremia after transsphenoidal surgery for pituitary adenomas. Endocrine 2018;62:333–9.
14. Robertson GL. Antidiuretic hormone. Normal and disordered function. Endocrinol Metab Clin North Am 2001;30:671–94, vii.
15. Loh JA, Verbalis JG. Disorders of water and salt metabolism associated with pituitary disease. Endocrinol Metab Clin North Am 2008;37:213–34, x.
16. Hannon MJ, Finucane FM, Sherlock M, et al. Clinical review: disorders of water homeostasis in neurosurgical patients. J Clin Endocrinol Metab 2012;97: 1423–33.
17. Kristof RA, Rother M, Neuloh G, et al. Incidence, clinical manifestations, and course of water and electrolyte metabolism disturbances following transsphenoidal pituitary adenoma surgery: a prospective observational study. J Neurosurg 2009;111: 555–62.
18. Sheehan JM, Sheehan JP, Douds GL, et al. DDAVP use in patients undergoing transsphenoidal surgery for pituitary adenomas. Acta Neurochir (Wien) 2006; 148:287–91 [discussion: 291].
19. Ajlan AM, Abdulqader SB, Achrol AS, et al. Diabetes insipidus following endoscopic transsphenoidal surgery for pituitary adenoma. J Neurol Surg B Skull Base 2018;79:117–22.
20. Broersen LHA, Biermasz NR, van Furth WR, et al. Endoscopic vs. microscopic transsphenoidal surgery for Cushing's disease: a systematic review and meta-analysis. Pituitary 2018;21(5):524–34.
21. Goudakos JK, Markou KD, Georgalas C. Endoscopic versus microscopic trans-sphenoidal pituitary surgery: a systematic review and meta-analysis. Clin Otolaryngol 2011;36:212–20.
22. Agam MS, Wedemeyer MA, Wrobel B, et al. Complications associated with microscopic and

endoscopic transsphenoidal pituitary surgery: experience of 1153 consecutive cases treated at a single tertiary care pituitary center. J Neurosurg 2018. [Epub ahead of print].

23. Akbari H, Malek M, Ghorbani M, et al. Clinical outcomes of endoscopic versus microscopic transsphenoidal surgery for large pituitary adenoma. Br J Neurosurg 2018;32:206–9.

24. Little AS, Kelly DF, White WL, et al. Results of a prospective multicenter controlled study comparing surgical outcomes of microscopic versus fully endoscopic transsphenoidal surgery for nonfunctioning pituitary adenomas: the Transsphenoidal Extent of Resection (TRANSSPHER) study. J Neurosurg 2019. [Epub ahead of print].

25. Wedemeyer MA, Lin M, Fredrickson VL, et al. Recurrent Rathke's cleft cysts: incidence and surgical management in a tertiary pituitary center over 2 decades. Oper Neurosurg (Hagerstown) 2018;16(6):675–84.

26. Hayashi Y, Aida Y, Sasagawa Y, et al. Delayed occurrence of diabetes insipidus after transsphenoidal surgery with radiologic evaluation of the pituitary stalk on magnetic resonance imaging. World Neurosurg 2018;110:e1072–7.

27. Faltado AL, Macalalad-Josue AA, Li RJS, et al. Factors associated with postoperative diabetes insipidus after pituitary surgery. Endocrinol Metab (Seoul) 2017;32:426–33.

28. Nemergut EC, Zuo Z, Jane JA Jr, et al. Predictors of diabetes insipidus after transsphenoidal surgery: a review of 881 patients. J Neurosurg 2005;103:448–54.

29. Sigounas DG, Sharpless JL, Cheng DM, et al. Predictors and incidence of central diabetes insipidus after endoscopic pituitary surgery. Neurosurgery 2008;62:71–8 [discussion: 78–9].

30. Hensen J, Henig A, Fahlbusch R, et al. Prevalence, predictors and patterns of postoperative polyuria and hyponatraemia in the immediate course after transsphenoidal surgery for pituitary adenomas. Clin Endocrinol (Oxf) 1999;50:431–9.

31. Olson BR, Rubino D, Gumowski J, et al. Isolated hyponatremia after transsphenoidal pituitary surgery. J Clin Endocrinol Metab 1995;80:85–91.

32. Casulari LA, Costa KN, Albuquerque RC, et al. Differential diagnosis and treatment of hyponatremia following pituitary surgery. J Neurosurg Sci 2004;48:11–8.

33. Barber SM, Liebelt BD, Baskin DS. Incidence, etiology and outcomes of hyponatremia after transsphenoidal surgery: experience with 344 consecutive patients at a single tertiary center. J Clin Med 2014;3:1199–219.

34. Williams CN, Riva-Cambrin J, Bratton SL. Etiology of postoperative hyponatremia following pediatric

35. Sata A, Hizuka N, Kawamata T, et al. Hyponatremia after transsphenoidal surgery for hypothalamo-pituitary tumors. Neuroendocrinology 2006;83:117–22.

36. Sane T, Rantakari K, Poranen A, et al. Hyponatremia after transsphenoidal surgery for pituitary tumors. J Clin Endocrinol Metab 1994;79:1395–8.

37. Boehnert M, Hensen J, Henig A, et al. Severe hyponatremia after transsphenoidal surgery for pituitary adenomas. Kidney Int Suppl 1998;64:S12–4.

38. Tymms J, Clark JD, Griffith HB, et al. Pituitary surgery and inappropriate antidiuretic hormone secretion. J R Soc Med 1992;85:302.

39. Little AS, Yuen K. Letter to the editor. Pituitary 2018;21:334.

40. Erkut ZA, Pool C, Swaab DF. Glucocorticoids suppress corticotropin-releasing hormone and vasopressin expression in human hypothalamic neurons. J Clin Endocrinol Metab 1998;83:2066–73.

41. Cole CD, Gottfried ON, Liu JK, et al. Hyponatremia in the neurosurgical patient: diagnosis and management. Neurosurg Focus 2004;16:E9.

42. Staiger RD, Sarnthein J, Wiesli P, et al. Prognostic factors for impaired plasma sodium homeostasis after transsphenoidal surgery. Br J Neurosurg 2013;27:63–8.

43. Verbalis JG, Goldsmith SR, Greenberg A, et al. Diagnosis, evaluation, and treatment of hyponatremia: expert panel recommendations. Am J Med 2013;126(10 Suppl 1):S1–42.

44. Verbalis JG. Management of disorders of water metabolism in patients with pituitary tumors. Pituitary 2002;5:119–32.

45. Hoorn EJ, Zietse R. Water balance disorders after neurosurgery: the triphasic response revisited. NDT Plus 2010;3:42–4.

46. Loh JA, Verbalis JG. Diabetes insipidus as a complication after pituitary surgery. Nat Clin Pract Endocrinol Metab 2007;3:489–94.

47. Seckl J, Dunger D. Postoperative diabetes insipidus. BMJ 1989;298:2–3.

48. Hans P, Stevenaert A, Albert A. Study of hypotonic polyuria after trans-sphenoidal pituitary adenomectomy. Intensive Care Med 1986;12:95–9.

49. Hoffman H, Ziechmann R, Gould G, et al. The impact of aneurysm location on incidence and etiology of hyponatremia following subarachnoid hemorrhage. World Neurosurg 2018;110:e621–6.

50. Kao L, Al-Lawati Z, Vavao J, et al. Prevalence and clinical demographics of cerebral salt wasting in patients with aneurysmal subarachnoid hemorrhage. Pituitary 2009;12:347–51.

51. Costa MM, Esteves C, Castedo JL, et al. A challenging coexistence of central diabetes

insipidus and cerebral salt wasting syndrome: a case report. J Med Case Rep 2018;12:212.

52. Momi J, Tang CM, Abcar AC, et al. Hyponatremia - what is cerebral salt wasting? Perm J 2010;14:62–5.

53. Yee AH, Burns JD, Wijdicks EF. Cerebral salt wasting: pathophysiology, diagnosis, and treatment. Neurosurg Clin N Am 2010;21:339–52.

54. Hannon MJ, Behan LA, O'Brien MM, et al. Hyponatremia following mild/moderate subarachnoid hemorrhage is due to SIAD and glucocorticoid deficiency and not cerebral salt wasting. J Clin Endocrinol Metab 2014;99:291–8.

55. Spasovski G, Vanholder R, Allolio B, et al, Hyponatraemia Guideline Development Group. Clinical practice guideline on diagnosis and treatment of hyponatraemia. Nephrol Dial Transplant 2014; 29(Suppl 2):i1–39.

56. Kinik ST, Kandemir N, Baykan A, et al. Fludrocortisone treatment in a child with severe cerebral salt wasting. Pediatr Neurosurg 2001;35:216–9.

57. Taplin CE, Cowell CT, Silink M, et al. Fludrocortisone therapy in cerebral salt wasting. Pediatrics 2006; 118:e1904–8.

58. Dumont AS, Nemergut EC 2nd, Jane JA Jr, et al. Postoperative care following pituitary surgery. J Intensive Care Med 2005;20:127–40.

59. Verbalis JG. Disorders of water metabolism: diabetes insipidus and the syndrome of inappropriate antidiuretic hormone secretion. Handb Clin Neurol 2014;124:37–52.

60. Nemergut EC, Dumont AS, Barry UT, et al. Perioperative management of patients undergoing transsphenoidal pituitary surgery. Anesth Analg 2005; 101:1170–81.

61. Ball SG, Vaidja B, Baylis PH. Hypothalamic adipsic syndrome: diagnosis and management. Clin Endocrinol (Oxf) 1997;47:405–9.

62. Vance ML. Perioperative management of patients undergoing pituitary surgery. Endocrinol Metab Clin North Am 2003;32:355–65.

63. Takeuchi K, Nagatani T, Okumura E, et al. A novel method for managing water and electrolyte balance after transsphenoidal surgery: preliminary study of moderate water intake restriction. Nagoya J Med Sci 2014;76:73–82.

64. Matsuyama J, Ikeda H, Sato S, et al. Early water intake restriction to prevent inappropriate antidiuretic hormone secretion following transsphenoidal surgery: low BMI predicts postoperative SIADH. Eur J Endocrinol 2014;171:711–6.

65. Lockett J, Berkman KE, Dimeski G, et al. Urea treatment in fluid restriction-refractory hyponatraemia. Clin Endocrinol (Oxf) 2019;90(4):630–6.

66. Olson BR, Gumowski J, Rubino D, et al. Pathophysiology of hyponatremia after transsphenoidal pituitary surgery. J Neurosurg 1997;87:499–507.

67. Zada G, Liu CY, Fishback D, et al. Recognition and management of delayed hyponatremia following transsphenoidal pituitary surgery. J Neurosurg 2007;106:66–71.

68. Wei T, Zuyuan R, Changbao S, et al. Hyponatremia after transspheniodal surgery of pituitary adenoma. Chin Med Sci J 2003;18:120–3.

69. Bohl MA, Ahmad S, White WL, et al. Implementation of a postoperative outpatient care pathway for delayed hyponatremia following transsphenoidal surgery. Neurosurgery 2018;82:110–7.

70. Hussain NS, Piper M, Ludlam WG, et al. Delayed postoperative hyponatremia after transsphenoidal surgery: prevalence and associated factors. J Neurosurg 2013;119:1453–60.

71. Jahangiri A, Wagner J, Tran MT, et al. Factors predicting postoperative hyponatremia and efficacy of hyponatremia management strategies after more than 1000 pituitary operations. J Neurosurg 2013; 119:1478–83.

1. Publication Title	2. Publication Number	3. Filing Date
NEUROSURGERY CLINICS OF NORTH AMERICA	0010 – 548	9/18/2019

4. Issue Frequency	5. Number of Issues Published Annually	6. Annual Subscription Price
JAN, APR, JUL, OCT	4	$430.00

7. Complete Mailing Address of Known Office of Publication *(Not printer) (Street, city, county, state, and ZIP+4®)*

ELSEVIER INC.
230 Park Avenue, Suite 800
New York, NY 10169

Contact Person
STEPHEN R. BUSHING

Telephone *(Include area code)*
215-239-3688

8. Complete Mailing Address of Headquarters or General Business Office of Publisher *(Not printer)*

ELSEVIER INC.
230 Park Avenue, Suite 800
New York, NY 10169

9. Full Names and Complete Mailing Addresses of Publisher, Editor, and Managing Editor *(Do not leave blank)*

Publisher *(Name and complete mailing address)*

TAYLOR BALL, ELSEVIER INC.
1600 JOHN F KENNEDY BLVD. SUITE 1800
PHILADELPHIA, PA 19103-2899

Editor *(Name and complete mailing address)*

STACY EASTMAN, ELSEVIER INC.
1600 JOHN F KENNEDY BLVD. SUITE 1800
PHILADELPHIA, PA 19103-2899

Managing Editor *(Name and complete mailing address)*

PATRICK MANLEY, ELSEVIER INC.
1600 JOHN F KENNEDY BLVD. SUITE 1800
PHILADELPHIA, PA 19103-2899

10. Owner *(Do not leave blank. If the publication is owned by a corporation, give the name and address of the corporation immediately followed by the names and addresses of all stockholders owning or holding 1 percent or more of the total amount of stock. If not owned by a corporation, give the names and addresses of the individual owners. If owned by a partnership or other unincorporated firm, give its name and address as well as those of each individual owner. If the publication is published by a nonprofit organization, give its name and address.)*

Full Name	Complete Mailing Address
WHOLLY OWNED SUBSIDIARY OF REED/ELSEVIER, US HOLDINGS	1600 JOHN F KENNEDY BLVD, SUITE 1800 PHILADELPHIA, PA 19103-2899

11. Known Bondholders, Mortgagees, and Other Security Holders Owning or Holding 1 Percent or More of Total Amount of Bonds, Mortgages, or Other Securities. If none, check box. ▶ ☐ None

Full Name	Complete Mailing Address
N/A	

12. Tax Status *(For completion by nonprofit organizations authorized to mail at nonprofit rates) (Check one)*
The purpose, function, and nonprofit status of this organization and the exempt status for federal income tax purposes:
☒ Has Not Changed During Preceding 12 Months
☐ Has Changed During Preceding 12 Months *(Publisher must submit explanation of change with this statement)*

PS Form **3526**, July 2014 *(Page 1 of 4 (see instructions page 4))* PSN: 7530-01-000-9931 PRIVACY NOTICE: See our privacy policy on www.usps.com.

13. Publication Title	14. Issue Date for Circulation Data Below
NEUROSURGERY CLINICS OF NORTH AMERICA	JULY 2019

15. Extent and Nature of Circulation		Average No. Copies Each Issue During Preceding 12 Months	No. Copies of Single Issue Published Nearest to Filing Date
a. Total Number of Copies *(Net press run)*		158	150
b. Paid Circulation *(By Mail and Outside the Mail)*	(1) Mailed Outside-County Paid Subscriptions Stated on PS Form 3541 *(Include paid distribution above nominal rate, advertiser's proof copies, and exchange copies)*	49	55
	(2) Mailed In-County Paid Subscriptions Stated on PS Form 3541 *(Include paid distribution above nominal rate, advertiser's proof copies, and exchange copies)*	0	0
	(3) Paid Distribution Outside the Mails Including Sales Through Dealers and Carriers, Street Vendors, Counter Sales, and Other Paid Distribution Outside USPS®	41	62
	(4) Paid Distribution by Other Classes of Mail Through the USPS *(e.g., First-Class Mail®)*	0	0
c. Total Paid Distribution *(Sum of 15b (1), (2), (3), and (4))*	▶	90	117
d. Free or Nominal Rate Distribution *(By Mail and Outside the Mail)*	(1) Free or Nominal Rate Outside-County Copies included on PS Form 3541	54	17
	(2) Free or Nominal Rate In-County Copies Included on PS Form 3541	0	0
	(3) Free or Nominal Rate Copies Mailed at Other Classes Through the USPS *(e.g., First-Class Mail)*	0	0
	(4) Free or Nominal Rate Distribution Outside the Mail *(Carriers or other means)*	0	0
e. Total Free or Nominal Rate Distribution *(Sum of 15d (1), (2), (3) and (4))*	▶	54	17
f. Total Distribution *(Sum of 15c and 15e)*	▶	144	134
g. Copies not Distributed *(See Instructions to Publishers #4 (page 43))*	▶	14	16
h. Total *(Sum of 15f and g)*	▶	158	150
i. Percent Paid *(15c divided by 15f times 100)*	▶	62.5%	87.31%

* If you are claiming electronic copies, go to line 16 on page 3. If you are not claiming electronic copies, skip to line 17 on page 3.

16. Electronic Copy Circulation	Average No. Copies Each Issue During Preceding 12 Months	No. Copies of Single Issue Published Nearest to Filing Date
a. Paid Electronic Copies ▶		
b. Total Paid Print Copies (Line 15c) + Paid Electronic Copies (Line 16a) ▶		
c. Total Print Distribution (Line 15f) + Paid Electronic Copies (Line 16a) ▶		
d. Percent Paid (Both Print & Electronic Copies) (16b divided by 16c × 100) ▶		

☐ I certify that 50% of all my distributed copies (electronic and print) are paid above a nominal price.

17. Publication of Statement of Ownership

☒ If the publication is a general publication, publication of this statement is required. Will be printed
in the OCTOBER 2019 issue of this publication.

☐ Publication not required.

18. Signature and Title of Editor, Publisher, Business Manager, or Owner

Stephen R. Bushing   Date 9/18/2019

STEPHEN R. BUSHING - INVENTORY DISTRIBUTION CONTROL MANAGER

I certify that all information furnished on this form is true and complete. I understand that anyone who furnishes false or misleading information on this form or who omits material or information requested on the form may be subject to criminal sanctions (including fines and imprisonment) and/or civil sanctions (including civil penalties).

PS Form **3526**, July 2014 *(Page 3 of 4)* PRIVACY NOTICE: See our privacy policy on www.usps.com

Moving?

Make sure your subscription moves with you!

To notify us of your new address, find your **Clinics Account Number** (located on your mailing label above your name), and contact customer service at:

Email: journalscustomerservice-usa@elsevier.com

800-654-2452 (subscribers in the U.S. & Canada)
314-447-8871 (subscribers outside of the U.S. & Canada)

Fax number: 314-447-8029

Elsevier Health Sciences Division
Subscription Customer Service
3251 Riverport Lane
Maryland Heights, MO 63043

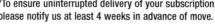

Printed and bound by CPI Group (UK) Ltd, Croydon, CR0 4YY

08/05/2025

01864745-0017